Endorsements

"This would be an inspiration for someone facing cancer."

– Sharon J, Pennsylvania

"I am not sure where to begin. I feel overwhelmed and speechless. I read everything without pausing for a moment because the more I read the more I was in awe. I chuckled, I cried, I cringed, I hurt, I smiled, I gasped, I shook my head, I felt paralyzed and overwhelmed yet so informed and so intrigued. This book will bring people hope and insight."

– Teresa M, New York

Sur5or:
My Story

JOANNE LONEGRO-BABBINO

BALBOA.
PRESS

A DIVISION OF HAY HOUSE

Balboa Press books may be ordered through booksellers or by contacting:

Balboa Press
A Division of Hay House
1663 Liberty Drive
Bloomington, IN 47403
www.balboapress.com
1 (877) 407-4847

Because of the dynamic nature of the Internet, any web addresses or links contained in this book may have changed since publication and may no longer be valid. The views expressed in this work are solely those of the author and do not necessarily reflect the views of the publisher, and the publisher hereby disclaims any responsibility for them.

The author of this book does not dispense medical advice or prescribe the use of any technique as a form of treatment for physical, emotional, or medical problems without the advice of a physician, either directly or indirectly. The intent of the author is only to offer information of a general nature to help you in your quest for emotional and spiritual well-being. In the event you use any of the information in this book for yourself, which is your constitutional right, the author and the publisher assume no responsibility for your actions.

Any people depicted in stock imagery provided by Thinkstock are models, and such images are being used for illustrative purposes only.
Certain stock imagery © Thinkstock.

Printed in the United States of America.

ISBN: 978-1-4525-9650-1 (sc)
ISBN: 978-1-4525-9652-5 (hc)
ISBN: 978-1-4525-9651-8 (e)

Library of Congress Control Number: 2014907325

Balboa Press rev. date: 4/25/2014

To my husband, John, and my daughters, Megan and Emma. They gave me something to fight for, and I want them to remember that life is always worth fighting for.

Contents

Acknowledgments

I want to thank my mom and dad for always being there for me. Their support over the years has been amazing, and it is always very much appreciated. I am blessed to have two parents as loving as they are!

I also want to thank my sister, my brother, and all of my family members and friends who supported me through this very tough battle. I appreciate each and every one of you so much.

2003

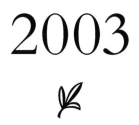

Chapter 1

"Normal" Life

Well let's see, it all began with a script for a baseline mammogram in the fall of 2003. I was thirty-seven years old. Yes, I know that a baseline mammogram is supposed to be taken at the age of thirty-five.

I was given a script for my baseline in late 2001, but I put it off. *There's no history of breast cancer in my family, I am not at risk; It's just a baseline; I've heard that it hurts,* and many other thoughts of this nature crossed my mind. Well, I put it off a little while longer, and then in the summer of 2002, I was pregnant with my second child. Megan, my oldest, was three and a half at the time. "Well, I can't do it now," I said to myself.

I had Emma in April 2003. I went for my ob-gyn checkup in the fall of 2003, and they mentioned that it looked like I never went for my baseline mammogram. They gave me a new script. I knew I had to make an appointment. But I waited—okay, procrastinated—yet again. My mom suggested a certain technician who used a heating pad to keep the x-ray unit nice and warm, and she said the technician was great. Apparently she was so great that I had to wait until January 14, 2004, to get an appointment with her. So I made my appointment and waited ...

I am the big planner and organizer of the family (just like my mother). So in June 2003, I started planning my sister's honeymoon cruise. She was getting married in April 2004. The people in the bridal party and a few friends were going to join her and her husband on their honeymoon cruise. I did all of the research and made the reservations for fourteen of us to fly down to San Juan and take a southern Caribbean cruise that went to Barbados, Aruba, Saint Thomas, and Dominica. I coordinated the entire vacation. Since the plans were being made so far in advance and we all had children, we all purchased trip insurance just in case. We were all psyched to get away together and couldn't wait for the big day.

In the mean-time, around October/November 2003, I got a call from a friend of mine with some not-so-good news. She had just been diagnosed with inflammatory breast cancer, which she said was technically stage IV.

I had never heard of this type of cancer before. She told me that since it's not as well known it is not usually diagnosed correctly, until it's too late. Instead of forming a lump, it starts off looking like an allergic reaction. The skin often looks like an orange rind, and the person is usually sent to a dermatologist to try skin remedies. When those don't work, they finally realize that it is cancer. Since it is a highly invasive and fast-spreading cancer they could not start with surgery because it would aggravate the cancer causing it to spread and then she would surely not survive. She told me she was going to have to have radiation, followed by a mastectomy, and then chemotherapy. As my friend started on her path of treatment, questions, and worries, I was very worried for her, because she had a daughter who was around the age of seven. Although we didn't live very close to each other anymore, I made sure that she knew that I was there for her for whatever she needed.

2004

Chapter 2

The Year I Would Like to Forget— The Beginning

On January 14, 2004, I went and had my mammogram. "Well, that's done. What a relief! It wasn't as bad as I thought it would be," I said to myself, and I ran off and did some errands. I got home about an hour or so later, and there was a message on my answering machine saying I needed to call the radiologist's office. For some reason, right at that moment, I felt my stomach drop. I had a really uneasy feeling about that message even though I am usually a glass-half-full type of person. Normally they send a letter in the mail. They don't call you right away unless something's up. When I returned the call, they said that since I was young, I had dense tissue and would need to make an appointment for additional mammograms and a sonogram. The first appointment available to do both procedures was not until a week later. Again I waited and I worried silently.

On Wednesday, January 21, 2004, I went for the additional mammograms and a sonogram. By that time I was a little amped up. I told the office personnel, the technician, and whoever else would listen that I was not leaving until I spoke to the doctor who read my films. I wanted to make sure that they got all the information they needed and that I found out what was going on. *I was not going to wait again!* The office manager seemed to understand my anxiety and assured me that I wouldn't leave without being informed.

I sat in the waiting room for a little while, and then they called my name to go into the office. The office manager took me back to see the radiologist. My heart was pounding. I just did not have a good feeling. I can't explain how I knew something was wrong; I just knew. The radiologist told me that in addition to some regular cysts, there was one lump in my right breast that didn't look like the others. The radiologist recommended that I get in contact with my ob-gyn and get a referral to a surgeon within the next couple of weeks. I responded that I was going to sit there and wait for copies of my films and then go directly to the ob-gyn. I was going to see a doctor, get a referral, and meet with a surgeon that same day! At that point, they probably thought I was slightly certifiable. But when someone gives you this type of information, do they realistically expect you to sit back and wait a couple of weeks? Really now!

They saw how upset I was, so they called my ob-gyn's office and told them to expect me. I called the office at the same time and told them that I wanted to see someone immediately. I can be a real bitch when I'm scared or threatened. Here I was going nuts all by myself. I was supposed to go back to work that afternoon, but I couldn't. I called my friend in the office, and she suggested I take the rest of that day and the next day off to get things in order. She said she would tell my boss what was going on.

I called my husband, John, to tell him what was going on. He was of the notion that until the doctors told us otherwise, everything was going to be fine. I tried to explain to him that I just *knew* something was wrong, but he said that we needed to wait and see for sure. There was no convincing him at this point.

I got my films and took off. I went directly to the ob-gyn. They were expecting me, of course. I spoke with the doctor and the nurse practitioner there. They got me in contact with a surgeon, but he only had office hours on Mondays and Fridays because he was in surgery the rest of the week so I scheduled an appointment for Friday … Then I had to wait for another day and a half, which was honestly one of the hardest things that I had ever had to do. I wanted to know now! I have a hard time with the unknown, as I'm sure most people do, and waiting in these types of situations is excruciating! It takes a toll on you mentally. Especially for a type "A" person who uses their brain a lot.

Something wasn't right. I knew it was bad. I don't know how, but I just knew. John was the optimistic one in this case. He said, "Everything is fine until they tell us otherwise." Yeah right, that was easy for him to say.

Chapter 3

The First Surgeon Visit

On Friday, January 23, 2004, John and I made the trip to the surgeon's office. I went in and met with the doctor. He examined the films and said it didn't look like a regular cyst, so he needed to take a core needle biopsy. He used a local anesthetic and then took three tissue samples. I asked him what would happen next. He told me that if the biopsy came back negative then he had missed. In other words, he knew that it was *cancer!*

Suddenly, at least a dozen things ran through my mind. I had a nine-month-old daughter and a five-year-old daughter who had mild cerebral palsy and wore braces on both of her legs. I had a full-time job. I had a husband who also worked full-time. I owned a house that I had to take care of. What was I going to do? Was I going to be there to watch my daughters grow up? Would I get to see them graduate, get married, or have kids? I couldn't breathe.

The next words I heard were, "Would you like us to go get your husband?"

I responded, "I don't know. Would you like a hole in your wall?" I don't know why that came out of my mouth. It was as if it wasn't me; it's hard to describe, but I'm sure many of you know exactly what I mean. I could literally visualize myself punching or kicking a hole in the office wall. I felt as if I was suffocating. One person stayed in the office with me while someone went to get John.

We then went in to the surgeon's office and spoke about next steps.

It was all such a blur. The surgeon told us that we needed to wait for the biopsy results but that they would try to put a rush on it. He explained that the lump he biopsied had certain characteristics that led him to believe that it was definitely cancer. We were to meet with him again when the results came back, in about a week. *Great*, I thought, *now I have to wait for the diagnosis to be officially confirmed.*

John and I decided to drive to my parents' house which was nearby and fill them in on all of this. We told them that the surgeon had essentially said that it was cancer and that the test was merely a formality. They took it very well and didn't get as upset as I had—at least not while I was there. My mom said that we would hit this thing head-on and go through all the steps to ensure that we got the cancer ("IT") out of my life as quickly as "IT" had arrived. We hugged each other and I said that I would keep them informed.

My parents shared the news with my sister and my brother. They were worried, and they wanted to know if I should get a second doctor's opinion. I assured them I was comfortable with the surgeon that I was already working with. He was from Europe and was educated there. I lived in Germany for a few years when I was younger and I liked the way medicine was approached there. The medical professionals were more open-minded and focused on root causes as opposed to treating symptoms. My surgeon also made me feel very comfortable and was easy to talk to, so I was going to stick with him. Ultimately it was my decision to make. You will soon see that many things are outside of one's control. When you come across things that are within your control or things you can change to be within your control, it is important and empowering to seize the opportunity and take control wherever and whenever you can!

Since the diagnosis was not confirmed, I only told a few people at work. My health situation felt very private, but when it appeared that my career might be affected, some discussions had to take place with a few people at work. It was very difficult to share the information without getting upset and crying.

Chapter 4

The Call

I got the call on Thursday, January 29 while I was at work. The surgeon spoke with me himself to say that it was indeed breast cancer, and we needed to come to the office the next day to start moving forward with treatment. I got upset and then called John and my parents to let them know. My parents were going to call the relatives on my side of the family. John called his mother and she said that she would call those on his side. I had to let a few more people at work know about my situation because they needed to know what my schedule would be, but it was really hard to say much. It was too new, too raw, and too scary! The few people I spoke to promised to keep it confidential and they did.

I couldn't talk about the fact that I had cancer without totally losing it. I constantly had a lump in my throat. It was hard to even say the word *cancer*. I had not been very sick in my life except for getting strep throat and ear infections when I was a kid. So this turn of events seemed crazy to me.

My dad was very upset. He felt that it wasn't fair, and I agreed. I had previously been married and cheated on, so I got divorced. I eventually got remarried. My older daughter was born at twenty-eight weeks, spent a month in NICU, and has cerebral palsy; my younger daughter was born at thirty-six weeks with a small hole in her heart, although it eventually closed. And now I was preparing to fight cancer? Hadn't I received more than my fair share of challenges?

Chapter 5

The Plan

When we returned to the surgeon's office after my diagnosis was confirmed, we scheduled the surgery for February 5, 2004, which was also my mom's birthday. It would be a lumpectomy and dissection of ancillary lymph nodes. Depending upon how I came out of surgery, I would either get to go home the same day or stay in the hospital overnight. I was mentally planning on going home the day of the surgery. My five-year-old, Megan, was very attached to me and wouldn't understand what was going on. I didn't know how to explain this to a five-year-old.

The surgeon explained that the type of dissection I was undergoing had a much lower chance of resulting in a condition called Lymphedema. This is a complication wherein the lymph fluid—that yellowy-clear stuff around a cut that helps it heal—gets into your arm and stays there, usually creating permanent swelling, because there are few or no lymph nodes to pump the fluid back out. Lymphedema is typically treated with compression therapy. The patient wears a compression sleeve on his or her arm to work against the fluid that is present. This condition can arise any time after the surgery, even years later, or it could never happen. From the point of the surgery on, my right arm could no longer be used for an intravenous needle, blood pressure cuff, or finger prick for blood tests. I would have to wear a medical ID bracelet to notify people of this condition and I was not happy about this at all. I thought they were so ugly. After the surgery there were additional precautions I had to take to improve my changes of not getting lymphedema. For example, I needed to avoid any punctures or scratches to the skin on my right arm. Therefore, I would need to wear thick (preferably leather) gloves when gardening or doing yard work. If I did break the skin, I needed to clean it thoroughly, use a cream like Neosporin on the cut, and keep it bandaged until it healed. I eventually found a more decorative medical alert bracelet online. If I had to wear it every day, then I wanted it to be pretty and have some "bling" on it. I ensured that it still had the necessary medical information as well as the red medical alert insignia.

The surgeon said that he would remove the lump and they would test for good margins to ensure that there was enough healthy tissue surrounding the actual tumor, an indication that they got it all. The test consists of putting different-colored dye on the different sides of the lump of tissue and tumor that they remove, freezing it, and then taking cross sections (very thin slices) and examining them under a microscope to confirm that there was sufficient healthy tissue surrounding the tumor. If for some reason the margins are not good and the tumor is too close to the edge of the lump of tissue, they would have to schedule a follow-up surgery to remove more tissue and perform additional tests. I told my doctor to make sure he took enough the first time because I wasn't planning on doing this again.

He told me he would also remove a scoop of lymph nodes from under my arm, as he felt there was at least one lymph node that was abnormally hard to the touch. If cancer moves from your breast into your lymph nodes, it starts at the bottom, moves up through the nodes, and then spreads up into the neck region. Because of this, lymph nodes are tested from the bottom up to determine the stage of the cancer.

My surgeon said that I would need to see an oncologist after surgery to discuss chemotherapy and radiation treatments. The actual treatment protocol would depend upon the outcome of the surgery. The surgeon explained that the oncologist would probably treat the cancer aggressively since I was young and otherwise healthy. He gave me the name of the oncologist that he usually worked with. He also called and spoke to him to let him know that I would be contacting him after my surgery.

Chapter 6

Sharing of the News

Between January 30 and February 4 only a select few were graced with the knowledge of my impending operation, as far as I was aware. Most everything seemed outside of my control, which I hated, as I am an absolute control freak. I spent a lot of time on the computer researching and running multiple scenarios through my head. I was exhausted. What if I didn't hammer out all of the possibilities? What if there was something I didn't think of? Fear of the unknown can be debilitating! This is a good example of the mental toll that I spoke about earlier.

I didn't tell everyone what was going on, but I had to call my closest friends to let them know. First, I called Andrea, who had been my friend since 1983 when we worked together at Mid Island Department Store, which is no longer around. She was shocked and concerned, as many people she knew had died from different forms of cancer. I told her that I was going to be fine. Andrea was confident that nothing bad was going to happen to me. She told me that she was not going to get upset, because she knew I would pull through it and be fine. Her home is about twenty minutes from mine (depending on Long Island traffic), so she soon volunteered her time, taking the girls off my hands and helping in other ways. She's an amazing woman, and I cherish our friendship immensely.

Next, I called Sharon. I met her when I lived in Pennsylvania from 1991 to 1993. We worked together in the audit department of Lebanon Valley National Bank, which has since been acquired by other financial institutions. She too was very upset and worried. She was supportive and also offered herself up for whatever I might need. Distance would make this a little more difficult, so she said that I could call her any hour of the day or night if I needed to talk to anyone. She too is an amazing friend, and I wouldn't trade her for anything.

My last call was to my dear friend Gihan, who lives in Germany. I met her when I lived there from 1988 to 1991. I had met someone at Hofstra University in the ROTC program where the United States Army paid for his education and he paid it back through service in United States Army. He was assigned to Frankfurt, Germany, so we decided to get married right out of college. In the end, it was not the correct choice for us because we didn't truly know each other, but that's a story for a different time.

Gihan and I became very good friends during the three years that I lived in Frankfurt, and we kept in contact the best we could after I came back to the United States. Email made staying in touch much easier. Even though we hadn't seen each other in over a decade at the time of my diagnosis, our friendship grew stronger over the years. She's the type of friend that you can feel deeply connected to even without a physical presence. We could go for months without talking to each other, but as soon as we did, it felt like we had just gotten together for tea the night before. When I called her, she was very upset about my news and wanted to hug me, which was impossible over the phone. She promised that she and all of her friends would send me positive energy so that I got through this challenging time.

I went to work as usual and tried to keep as normal of a routine as possible for my daughters. Sometimes I cried for no reason (well as you might imagine, it wasn't really for no reason). I kept pretty much to myself. I didn't want to talk to anyone about my changing reality until I had to. I was inside my head, which isn't a great place to be—it can get very loud in there.

Chapter 7

The Surgery

When I left work on February 4, I felt very emotional. I was really scared about the very real, very close future. The team I worked with was and is amazing. We care so much about each other that our relationships have become quite personal. The select few and I were teary-eyed when I left the office, and I let them know that it was okay for them to share with the others in the office what was going on. It was much too difficult for me to repeat the story without getting upset, which would in turn get the other person upset.

I took my first of two sick days on February 5. Yes you read that correctly. John and I got the girls off to school and day care and then drove to the ambulatory surgery unit next to the hospital. I signed in, changed into the lovely hospital gown, and bagged up my belongings. The staff eventually came in and took my vitals.

I was very apprehensive about the IV being put in. Ever since I got mononucleosis in college and the people in the infirmary couldn't draw blood effectively, and made me feel like a human pincushion, I can't stand needles. I was black and blue down an entire arm. However, for this surgery, a nurse with an amazing reputation was recommended to me. When she inserted the IV, it went in much better than I expected. Then we waited.

My surgery was scheduled for 10:00 a.m., but I didn't get taken into the operating room until after 4:00 p.m. I was starving, and hence my mood worsened as the day progressed. I don't really recall being in recovery or being moved back to the ambulatory staging area, but I sort of remember speaking to the surgeon. I also remember seeing him sitting across the room at the nurse's desk, albeit he looked a little blurry from where I was laying. I ate crackers and drank some juice, and the next thing I knew, they told me that I needed to decide right away whether I was going to go home or stay overnight because the ambulatory surgery center would be closing soon.

I wanted to go home, and I was planning to go home, but I was in a good amount of pain, and my mom told me that I looked white as a sheet. I begrudgingly decided that I should stay overnight, so I was moved to a room in the hospital. I was fine until I stood up, and then my head spun and my stomach churned, and I proceeded to get sick as a dog. I was also in worse pain than before. At this point, morphine is your friend. I got one shot of it to carry me through the night. The nurse and I spoke, and we decided to change to a different pain medication so that I would be able to go home the next day—you are not allowed to go home with morphine in your system.

On the morning of February 6, I promptly got out of bed and washed my hair in the sink and did my makeup. There was a tube sticking out of my armpit attached to a little bulb slowly filling with lymph fluid. The surgeon came in and checked on me and explained that the plastic bulb had to be emptied twice a day by John. I also needed to keep an ace bandage wrapped tightly around my body; the tube for the drain was fastened to the bandage with a safety pin. I couldn't take a shower for the next few days or get the area wet. I mentioned that I had gotten sick, and he said that the anesthesiologist could give me an anti-nausea medication prior to any future surgeries. I thought that was a cool idea. I hated throwing up all over the place. It's just not very lady-like.

My follow-up appointment with the surgeon was scheduled for Monday, February 9. I was very stiff for the next few days. I didn't sleep very well because every time I rolled onto my right side out of habit, I woke up in pain. When I went to my follow-up appointment, the wound was still draining too much. The surgeon said that we couldn't leave it in much longer though, because my skin would start to grow onto it and then it would be more difficult and painful to remove. The surgeon cleared me to make an appointment with the oncologist, so I scheduled one for February 20, 2004.

I worked from home that week. Luckily, I could connect to my company's servers via VPN. As I think back, I remember being so grateful to have had the ability to continue to work. Working allowed me to concentrate on something other than my cancer, even if it was for short periods of time. I wonder if the whole situation might have turned out differently if I had not worked as I recovered and went through treatment.

On February 11, I went to have the surgeon check the drainage again. He said that although some liquid was still draining, the volume was much lower, and he had to remove the drain. He told me to take a deep breath, and then he pulled it out. Holy crap did it smart! He said that if the lymph fluid began to pool in my armpit, he would have to drain it with a needle. I saw the surgeon again the following week, and everything was progressing fine. We didn't have to do any manual drainage of lymph fluid, thank goodness.

I went back into the office for work the week of February 16. Everyone was very supportive, wished me well, and did not pry too much. Because of my type "A" personality, I need to be going one hundred miles per hour at all times, so I have to repeat how grateful I am that I was physically able to work. The word "relax" was not in my vocabulary then, and even now I have to be reminded to do so.

Chapter 8

The First Oncology Visit

My mom went with me to the oncologist's office on February 20, 2004, as John had to work. I brought my salt-and-pepper notebook full of questions, prepared to write things down when we spoke with the doctor. If this situation ever happens to you, and I hope it does not—make sure that you document everything and keep it organized throughout the process. There's so much going on in your mind and it is very easy to get confused. In addition, if you have children, it is helpful for them to have access to the documentation as part of their family medical history when they get older.

The waiting room for the oncology department was large. There was a big flat-screen television and a lot of magazines to read, but you knew why most people were there, and it is sort of depressing to realize that there is so much cancer out there.

One of the assistants called my name and my mom and I were taken to the oncologist's office. As I looked around the office waiting for him to walk in, I saw many plaques hanging on the wall, displaying his degrees, certifications, awards, and affiliations. When he introduced himself, he seemed very nice. I remember him saying that he would always tell me the truth, and I needed to trust him on that. He also told me that he wouldn't treat me any differently than he would his wife or daughter. If for some reason he was not as jovial, I should not think that it had anything to do with me, my condition, or my treatment. He explained that he had many other patients and could be reacting to elements other than me. He reiterated that if there was something that he needed to say to me about my condition or my treatment that he would. I got a good feeling about him, just like I had when I met the surgeon.

We discussed my diagnosis in light of the surgical results. He told me that I had infiltrating ductal carcinoma. The tumor was 3.2 centimeters wide, and three out of sixteen lymph nodes were involved, meaning they were positive for cancer. They were grade two cells—slow growing.

The oncologist explained that he was going to treat the cancer aggressively because I was so young and healthy, just like the surgeon had said. He told us that seventy-year-old women had undergone this same treatment with flying colors, so I should have no problem. I asked why the treatment would be so aggressive if the cancer cells were a slow-growing type. The oncologist responded that the more aggressive the treatment was, the greater the benefits were in reducing the chance of recurrence. I swallowed hard when I heard that word. I thought *I have to go through all of this crap now. Do you really think I am going to go through it again?* I know that many people experience cancer more than once in their life, but I was and still am very confident that this is not going to happen to me.

Next, the oncologist said that I needed to have a battery of tests prior to starting my chemotherapy treatment: a MUGA (cardiac test to check that my heart muscle was working well, as some of the chemicals can affect the heart); a CAT scan of my chest, abdomen, and pelvis with IV contrast (to make sure that my organs were all the correct size and that there was no signs of cancer); and a bone scan with an injection of radioactive material to rule out metastatic bone disease—in other words, to make sure the cancer was not in my bones.

I was told that at each visit, they would weigh me and track my red blood cells, white blood cells, platelets, and so on, to ensure that my body was well enough to handle the chemotherapy treatment. Therefore, I would have a finger stick (blood test) done prior to each treatment and between each treatment to ensure that my body was bouncing back.

He went on to discuss the protocol (a.k.a. treatment plan) in greater detail and provided me with drug information sheets. This next part gets a little technical. The first part of the protocol is a mixture of Cytoxan and Adriamycin, the drugs that can affect the heart, as well as Decadron. I would have four of these treatments over eight weeks: one week on, one week off. Before each treatment, they would give me Pepcid to soothe my stomach and Benadryl to reduce allergic reactions or itching. They would also give me an anti-nausea medication that was time-released over approximately five days. The treatment could cause nausea after the medication wore off as well as diarrhea and or constipation. Chemotherapy could lower the number of white blood cells and increase my chances of getting an infection. My number of platelets, which are necessary for proper blood clotting, could also drop. I would have to be careful while brushing my teeth, shaving my legs, etcetera. Twenty-four hours after the treatment, I would have to return to the office for a shot of Neulastin—an injection to boost my immune system since the chemo attacked my immune system and killed white blood cells to target any cancer cells in my body. This shot could cause bone pain, joint pain, and more, but it was necessary because it helped manage the chemo's effects on my immune system. They told me I could expect hair loss in three to four weeks after the first treatment, so I should procure a wig before that time. Sounds like a blast, right?

The second part of the protocol was Taxotere. We had two options: four treatments over eight weeks (one week on, one week off) like the first part of the protocol or twelve doses over fourteen weeks (four weeks on, one week off). This treatment, regardless of the timing, could affect my finger-nail color or cause nail loss altogether. The possibility of hair loss, nausea, body aches, bone pain, diarrhea, and constipation would continue. I would have to take Dexamethasone tablets the day before and after the Taxotere treatment to help offset the potential of severe fluid retention. The oncologist said that most people tolerate Taxotere better in smaller doses over a longer time period, so that was the route we should take. I agreed with him due to his vast experience.

The third part of the protocol was radiation therapy, five days a week for six weeks. This would be done at their corresponding radiological center and had its own set of possible side effects like fatigue, burned or irritated skin, and possible temporary diminished lung capacity.

The fourth part of protocol could include long-term hormone medication (like Tamoxifen) depending upon the findings of the tumor testing, which the oncologist hadn't received as of this appointment.

I thought: *What lovely potential side effects.* He mentioned that not everyone's experience is the same. He encouraged me to drink a lot of water to flush the chemo through my system as quickly as possible. The oncologist gave me a prescription for a wig so that it would potentially be covered by my health insurance.

Everything was so over-whelming and scary. I don't think the part about the hair loss hit me at the time. However, my mom made sure that I remained energized to get through this crap, beat "IT", and move on with my life.

After describing the course of treatment, the oncologist asked if I would have family support, as I was going to need it. At the time, my children were five years and nine months old. I was fortunate to report that I would have a lot of family around me: my husband; my parents, who live less than ten minutes away; my brother and his wife, who are at about the same distance; and my sister and her family, who are about twenty minutes away.

I then asked about whether I would still be able to go on my sister's honeymoon cruise in April. I bet you can guess what the answer was: no cruise! I was devastated. The doctor explained that because I would be in the middle of treatment, there was no way that I could go. And it would not be wise to put off the course of chemotherapy, because early detection and treatment are very important when dealing with cancer. He offered to provide me with whatever documentation I needed to cancel my cruise reservation without a financial penalty. Even so, I felt again like I was not in control. The disease was forcing me on a detour from my plans—my life. I dreaded telling my sister that even though I had planned the whole trip, I was not going to be able to go.

I asked how the oncologist felt about holistic treatment in conjunction with traditional treatment. He said that it would probably not be an issue, but I needed to send him a list of the supplements I planned to take so that he could check with the nutritionist on staff before I started.

After discussing all of this, I asked about a Life Port. My friend who was a couple of months ahead of me on this journey battling inflammatory breast cancer, had advised me that this was the way to go. The chemicals they inject through an IV can really damage your veins, and if your veins fail, the chemicals could leak into your body. Because my therapy would take many treatments and I could not use the veins in my right arm because of the risk of getting lymphedema, I figured that I should ask about this option. My oncologist was in favor of a port (also called a portacath) and said I should contact the surgeon to get it done as soon as possible.

A surgeon typically implants a port under the patient's skin in either the arm or chest area. A soft, slim tube connects to the port and goes through the chosen vein all the way to your heart. The catheter therefore protects the vein during treatment. Nurses can find it easily and use it for drawing blood as well as administering the treatment. For chemotherapy a nurse uses a special type of needle to access the port rather than hunting for a good vein. The benefits were reason enough for me to proceed with the implantation of the port. I was instructed not to let anyone other than the nurses access my port at the oncologist's office. They were trained in how to use one, and we did not want to risk infection by someone not treating it properly.

Before leaving the oncologist that day, we discussed the timing of my treatments. He said that I could choose whether I wanted to have my treatments on Mondays or Fridays. I chose Fridays because I figured I'd have the weekend to recuperate before work the next Monday, and I'd have family and friends to help with the girls over the weekend if I needed then. He said that my first treatment would be on February 27 one week later. This didn't give me much time to get all my tests done and my port implanted. It also meant that I'd probably lose my hair in less than a month. Oh joy!

I went home and called the radiologist to set up appointments for the required tests, but I found out that the radiology offices were not equipped to administer all of the necessary tests in one location. Here were more challenges I had to face, but it made me stronger in the end, right?

Prior to my cancer, Emma, my younger daughter, had a series of ear infections for about six months. As soon as she was off the antibiotics for one infection, she got another. And when she was sick, she didn't want anyone but me to care for her. It was exhausting for the whole family.

I knew that if this continued, it was going to be a problem once I started treatment. But because I experienced ear infections as a child and Megan had tubes put in her ears a few times due to chronic ear infections, John and I made the tough decision to have tubes put in Emma's ears as well. So, between all of my appointments, we squeezed in this procedure. Emma was a much happier baby after the surgery.

Chapter 9

The Hair, Part I

Next, I called my insurance company. I found out that everything regarding my treatment for breast cancer would be covered except for the wig, because it was considered to be for cosmetic purposes. I explained that I needed a wig because the chemotherapy was going to make my hair fall out and I even mentioned my prescription. However, the insurance company still said it would not be covered.

I started researching how much a wig would cost and found out that it depended upon whether it was synthetic or made with real hair. Wigs could run anywhere from forty dollars to a couple of thousand dollars. I was very torn on what to do because I didn't want it to be obvious I was wearing a wig, but I wasn't sure I wanted to pay for the best-looking options.

I decided to go see my hairdresser, Sal, who had been doing my hair since 1983. He was amazing. After I filled him in, Sal and I sat and talked about this new challenge in my life and all of my options. We decided to go with a real-hair wig because it would look the most natural, and I would have the flexibility to cut, color, and use a hairdryer to change it up if I felt like it. He and I joked that this would be the perfect time for me to experiment with a new look. Maybe I should go blonde or become a red-head like my sister. I decided to stick with my natural color, so I gave him a few pieces of my hair that he could use to find a wig color that matched as closely as possible. He ordered the wig from a company in Florida and only charged me for its cost and not the labor involved in customizing it. We women love our hair-dressers for very good reasons!

Soon afterward, I looked through a catalog to find a medical alert bracelet so that if I was ever in an emergency, people would know not to use my right arm for an IV insertion, finger stick, or blood pressure check. As I looked through the catalog, I decided to also order a long red-haired wig for Megan. I thought it would be fun for both of us to have new hair. I also wanted to make light of the fact that I would lose my hair so that it wouldn't be too scary for her.

I had a great support system. Although my struggle with cancer was a very private thing to go through, my aunts, cousins, friends, and husbands' friends all wanted to help. When they found out that the wig was not covered by insurance, unbeknownst to me, my aunt Santa (her real name) started a wig fund for me. My wonderful family and friends donated a total of $1,586, and the donations came with amazing notes of encouragement.

March 2, 2004

Santa,

Enclosed is a check for the Joanne fund. I did let the people, who are closed to her, at work know about the fund and I will forward anything I receive.

Please let Joanne know that we love her and to stay strong....

If there is anything else I can do please let me know. I can be reached at 631-███████

Hi Santa,

My name is Joe Fitzpatrick I am a friend of John Babbino's When I heard that family and friends were getting up a collection for Joanne, I told John that I would send a little something so Joanne and he could have a night out maybe dinner and a movie or something.

It is through tough times that family and friends make all the difference in the world, and help comfort each other.

I appreciate your help in getting this to Joanne and John. Thank You.

Dear Santa,

Jenny & I are enclosing a check for Joanne's "wig fund". The meaning of the amount of the check is enclosed.

Chai

This symbol, commonly seen on necklaces and other jewelry and ornaments, is simply the Hebrew word Chai (living), with the two Hebrew letters Chet and Yod attached to each other. Some say it refers to the Living God. Judaism as a religion is very focused on life, and the word chai has great significance. The typical Jewish toast is l'chayim (to life). Gifts to charity are routinely given in multiples of 18 (the numeric value of the word Chai).

to help keep Joanne beautiful.
Love,
Andrea

We just wanted to wish you and your family all the best. You are all in our thoughts.

We also wanted to send a little something to add to the collection you have going for Joanne's wig.

Tell the family we said hello and we look forward to meeting them the next time we visit New York!

Wig Fund – Notes of Support

1/31/04

Dear JoAnn,

Thank you for all your support to Berri, Brendon & family, over the years during our up or joyous occasions, and especially during our traumatic ordeals.

Please accept my sincere comments, as I would like to be here for you, as you fight with the sudden & terrible news of this type of illness.

The book on the subject of "Cancer" was purchased because, my mom, and others in my family have been thru this. My sister is a breast Ca survivor. These events have caused me to have a real passion for the quest of insight into the "Why?" of Ca., as well as "what can we do to survive it."

Some "Medical Doctors" also see the need of incorporating "Alternative scientifically proven remedy", as well as well as the benefit of chemo, & surgery.

So, I'm hoping to share a certain type of empowerment & confidence to give you more of a choice in the decision making process.

Do to the many different questions that may arise, of course its a lot to think about, never hurts to have the many experts research as possible. Please feel free to call on me at time, it would be an honor to assist you in any way. From my heart to yours, Carolyn

Support Letter

Chapter 10

More Gifts

When I was pregnant with Emma, I had to take it easy at twenty-eight weeks, because my water broke at twenty-eight weeks with Megan, and the doctor didn't know why. My sister and brother tried to convince me to hire someone to clean my house during this time. But we weren't brought up with a house-keeper, and I wasn't comfortable with having someone else clean my home. What if they didn't do it the way I did or the house wasn't as clean as when I did it? So I declined this recommendation.

When my sister, her husband, my brother, and his wife found out that I was sick, they all went behind my back and chipped in to hire someone named Eddy to clean for me. My siblings knew that if they asked me about it, I would refuse like I had before.

Eddy came to my house every other week to help me stay sane and not worry about keeping my house clean while I underwent treatment. Despite my initial resistance, it was the best gift anyone could ever give to someone with a type "A" personality like me. Before I was sick, I never really had three or four hours to clean my house anyway. I loved this gift so much that I decided to keep my house-keeper even after I was finished with my treatment.

Some of our friends gave us gift certificates to restaurants so that we could take a break from cooking when we wanted to. When I didn't feel like eating, John could go out and get some food and not have to cook for just Megan and him.

My mom started secretly making me a quilt—she's so lovingly sneaky like that. She sent fabric hearts and markers to my family and friends so that they could write supportive messages. She later collected these hearts and put them together in a very colorful, beautiful quilt. Every time I went to my treatments and pulled the quilt out, I got such wonderful compliments from the nurses and other patients. It was so bright that no one could miss it. I brought it to all of my chemotherapy appointments because we read that your body could feel cold. Whenever that happened, I had my positive energy blanket to cuddle up under, and I felt the love from my family and friends.

Here's the front of my quilt:

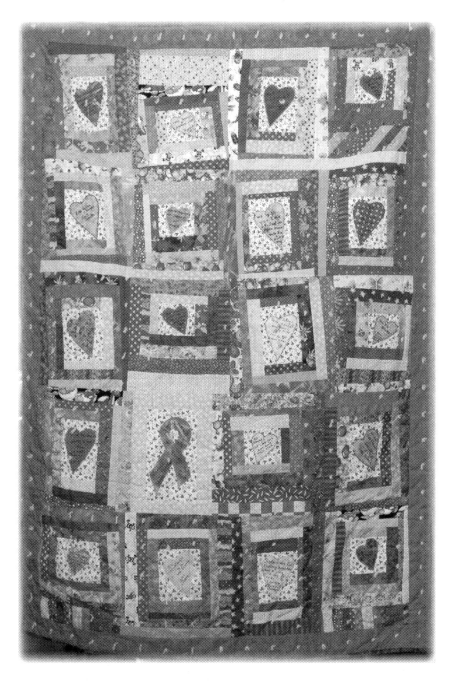

My Mom's Signature:

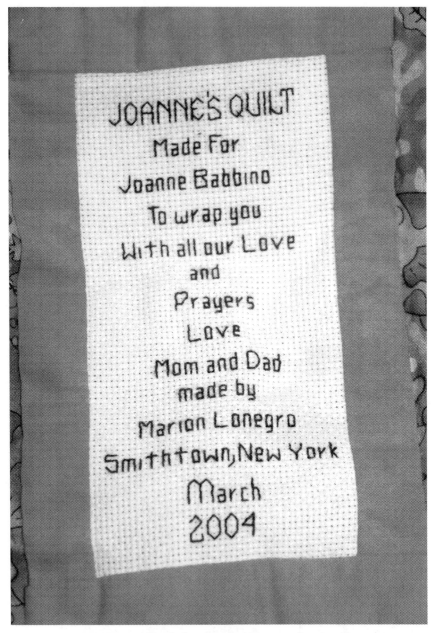

See Appendix A for more pictures of my quilt.

Chapter 11

The Administrative Nightmare—
Tests, Tasks, and More Surgery

On the morning of February 23, I had another appointment with the surgeon to check whether there was any lymph fluid building up in my armpit or arm. All looked well, and his bed-side manner and tone of voice always made me feel comfortable.

Later that morning, I had my bone scan. They injected me with a radioactive material, and then I had to go back three hours later and lay completely still for what felt like forever while they did the total body scan to see if there was any cancer in my bones.

In the downtime between the injection and the scan, I contacted the travel agent and told her that I wasn't going to be able to go on the cruise. She was very nice when I told her I had to cancel because I would be in treatments for my breast cancer. She got very quiet on the other end of the line and then said that she was so sorry. I thanked her and said that I was going to be fine, but I needed to take care of this. She understood and asked me to fax to her a cancellation request, which I did the same day. A few days, later I received confirmation that my reservation was indeed cancelled (a very sad day), but the cruise line had assessed a five-hundred-dollar cancellation penalty. I wasn't overly concerned though, because we had the trip insurance mentioned previously. I knew that my reasons for cancellation would be covered and I would get a full refund. I called the travel insurance company and again explained the situation. It was getting a little easier to talk about my situation now, at least with strangers. They told me that John needed to submit the cancellation request, stating that due to my illness, we would not be able to go. They would send us the forms to complete and submit with a physician statement form.

I called the airline, and they too said that I needed a letter from my doctor in order to cancel the reservation and get a refund without incurring a penalty, as the tickets we had purchased were technically not refundable. The lady I spoke to was originally going to give me a credit, but it would need to be used within a year. She said that if we didn't know when I'd actually be able to travel again, I should make sure that the letter from the doctor specifically stated that I would not be able to travel for at least one year. This way, I would be guaranteed a refund. I thanked her for all of her help. I was finding out that the kindness of strangers at convenient times was absolutely wonderful.

I told the representatives at both companies that I was going to see the oncologist on February 27, so I would get the letters and submit all the necessary paperwork at that point.

After my bone scan, I had my MUGA test the same afternoon. The technician injected me with some more radioactive material to identify my red blood cells and track them through my heart to make sure that the muscle walls were in normal working order.

The surgeon put in my port two days later, on February 25, 2004 at the ambulatory surgery center. My dad brought me to this appointment because John had to work that day, and we decided if he got the girls ready for the day their routine would be as normal as possible. When it was time for the IV to be put in, I strongly requested the same nurse from my lumpectomy. I think this upset the nurse who was working with me at the time, but I didn't care. I hate needles, and the other nurse had done a great job, and this in turn alleviated some of my anxiety. My dad stayed for a while and walked me in to surgery. I remembered to ask the anesthesiologist about anti-nausea medication, and he said that it would not be a problem.

The surgery schedule was running later than expected again, and my dad had another commitment, so he left and my aunt Santa came to take me home after the surgery. John was able to leave work and to pick up the girls from school and day care. When I got out of the surgery, I felt okay, not great. On the plus side, I didn't get physically ill, and the surgeon said it went well. I was in some amount of pain, but I didn't want to take pain medication. If I did, per hospital rules, I would have had to stay another hour prior to release, and I wanted to get home. My sister offered to watch the girls for John so that he could come get me, but my aunt was already there. Ultimately, John met us at the hospital to grab the prescription for pain medication and get it filled so that I could take it as soon as I got home.

By the time I got home and into bed, the pain was excruciating. It felt like I had been kicked in the shoulder by a horse. As I lay in bed crying hysterically, I thought: *If this is only the beginning and it's this bad, I don't think I want to or even can go through with this.* I was scared and emotional, and I just wanted to disappear. I wasn't thinking about my family; I was concentrating on my own mortality and my fears about what lay ahead. Before the surgery, I didn't realize that when they put in the port, they have to move things out of the way inside your body to install it. That is why the pain was so intense.

I was very tired and felt like crap. Megan, my five-year-old, sat in the bed next to me and said, "It's all right if you are tired, Mommy. I can keep you company and read to you." She was so adorable and caring that I wanted to cry more. Emma, my nine-month-old, was either sleeping or being watched by John at the time.

Megan even made me a card.

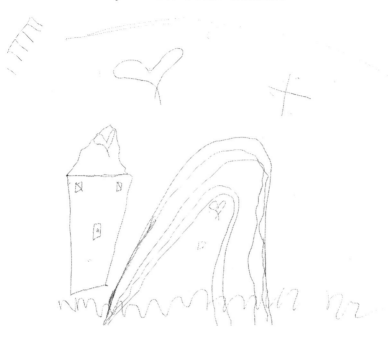

John had a lot thrust upon his shoulders during this time. He had to become even more involved with taking care of the girls. He stepped up without faltering and I was very thankful.

The next morning, February 26, I felt a little better and had to go in for my CAT scan. Prior to the test, I had to drink two bottles of liquid that I had picked up ahead of time. I drove myself to the test. This was when I realized that the portacath makes a lump under your skin right where the seat belt rests between your neck and your shoulder. It was very uncomfortable for about the first week.

Prior to starting the CAT scan, the technician explained that they would inject me with the contrast dye, and I would sense a warm feeling in the lower portion of my body. I also would feel sick to my stomach for a few moments, and then I would feel like I had to urinate. Some people have a reaction to the contrast dye, and they told me I should let the technician know if I got itchy. We worked through the list of known side effects and then proceeded with the test.

Toward the end, I started to get itchy. I mentioned it, and the technician said that some itching can be normal. However, I got itchier, and hives popped up. The test ended, and they looked at my skin. Lo and behold, I found out that I was allergic to the contrast dye. Because I had driven myself, they were hesitant to give me Benadryl, as it can make you sleepy. I told them that I usually took two when needed at home, and if they gave me one tablet, I would be fine. They agreed, but I had to wait to see how I reacted and whether I improved prior to getting sent home. In the future, I'll need to remember that I need to have steroids to counter-act my allergic reaction to the contrast dye used for a CAT scan.

Chapter 12

The First Chemotherapy Appointment

On the morning of February 27, I worked from home for a few hours. My first chemotherapy appointment was at 11:00 a.m. John took me, and we were both a little nervous.

We sat in the big waiting room and, well, waited. When they called my name, I went to the lab and got my finger stick done, as described previously. They also kept track of my weight. I had started dieting and exercising in the fall of 2003, before my diagnosis, and I had been successfully losing weight. I hoped to keep that trend going during the treatment even though I had heard that some people gain weight from steroids and the overall treatment protocol. However, I wanted something else that was in my control, so I always got excited for my weigh-ins.

At each appointment, the oncologist also checked my CBC (complete blood count) to detect the possible presence of anemia or infection and to determine how my body was reacting to the treatment. Listed below are the many items that they monitored, with the normal range as defined by the facility where I received treatment, along with the probable reasons why they monitored them (which I found out through doing further research).

Blood Smear—this is done to check the quantity, size, and shape of red blood cells, white blood cells, and platelets to ensure the patient has no blood diseases.

WBC—white blood cells (4.6–10.2): These cells (also called leukocytes) protect the body against infection. They are bigger in size and fewer in quantity than red blood cells. The number can be used to identify an infection or monitor the body's response to cancer treatment.

RBC—red blood cells (4.04–5.48): Red blood cells carry oxygen from the lungs to the rest of the body. If the count is low, the body may not be getting the oxygen it needs. This can cause fatigue, called anemia. Conversely, if the count is too high, there is a risk that the red blood cells will clump together and block tiny blood vessels. A high count can also indicate dehydration.

HGB—hemoglobin (12.2–16.2): Hemoglobin is the major substance in a red blood cell. The amount of hemoglobin is a good indication of the blood's ability to carry oxygen throughout the body. A higher than normal count could indicate dehydration.

HCT—hematocrit (37.7–47.9): This test measures the volume occupied by red blood cells—that is, the percentage of the blood that is made up of these cells. If the number is too high, it can also be another indication of dehydration.

These next four tests help in the diagnosis of different types of anemia.

MCV—mean corpuscular volume (80 – 97): This one shows the size of the red blood cells. A high volume count could indicate a lack of folic acid or vitamin B12, causing anemia. A low count can indicate anemia caused by a lack of iron.

MCH—mean corpuscular hemoglobin (27.0–31.2): This test shows the amount of hemoglobin in an average red blood cell.

MCHC—mean corpuscular hemoglobin concentration (31.8–35.4): This evaluation measures the concentration of hemoglobin in an average red blood cell. A low count can indicate anemia.

RDW—red cell distribution width (11.6–14.8): The RDW reports whether all the red cells are about the same width, size, and shape. This test helps further classify the different type of anemia a person might have.

PLT—platelet counts (142–424): Platelets are the smallest type of blood cell, and they play a major role in blood clotting. When bleeding occurs, the platelets swell, clump together, and form a sticky plug in the wound. A low number of platelets can be caused by infection or a lack of vitamin B12 or folic acid. If there are too few platelets, clotting may not occur to prevent excessive bleeding. A high number of platelets can be caused by many things, including infection or an iron deficiency. It also raises the risk of blood clots forming.

The other items on the card showing test results were labeled LYMPH, MPV, and GRAN. Aside from the first, I am not sure what was being measured by each.

I share all this technical information to illustrate that when I went through this experience, I wanted to know what they were monitoring and why as well as whether there was anything that I could do to keep my numbers in the good range.

After the blood work, I sat with the oncologist and mentioned the letter I needed in order to get a full refund from the airline. He dictated it right away and said that I could pick it up at my next appointment. My oncologist was very accommodating and helped me however he could.

He also signed the medical form to waive the cancellation penalty for the cruise. When I told him about the insurance company not covering the wig, he said he would work on it, but he did not think he could get that changed. I did not know yet at the time that my family was collecting a wig fund for me.

I had a lot of questions written down to ask my oncologist at this appointment. First, I asked him if I was allowed to take over-the-counter medicines, such as Tums for my stomach, cough drops, and vitamins including vitamin C supplements. He explained that I could not have vitamins the day before, day of, or day after a chemotherapy treatment and I could not take vitamin C at all, as it would counter-act the treatment.

I asked if I should have anti-nausea medicine at home, and he said that I shouldn't need it because the protocol that I was on included a time-released version. However, he told me that if I experienced any nausea, he could prescribe something.

I asked if there would be any memory issues, and I honestly don't remember what his answer was. I can tell you now that yes, there are memory issues—it is called chemo brain. I will get into this some more later on, if I can remember.

He said that fatigue could happen but usually intermittently, and there were medications to counteract it.

I also asked if we were going for a cure or regression. He explained that without treatment, there's a fifty percent chance of the cancer coming back, and his goal was to reduce this chance to somewhere in the range of twenty to twenty-five percent.

When I asked what stage of cancer I had, he said it was stage II. *Well, I guess that's good,* I thought. I figured that it put me in the middle as far as the severity of the disease.

By this appointment, the results of the testing on the tumor were back and we had some good news: it was estrogen-receptor negative. In other words, because the tumor was not estrogen based, I would not have to take the drug Tamoxifen. There are some potential long-term issues with this drug like the risk of developing other forms of cancer. The tumor was also progesterone-negative and HER2-negative. Because all of those markers were negative, one additional test called FISH (fluorescence in situ hybridization) was recommended to ensure that the review was complete. However, these results meant that I would not have to take any ongoing medication after my chemotherapy and radiation treatments were completed. I was very happy about that.

I asked about cancer markers—what they are, when they are done, and so forth. He said my markers were fine, but he didn't rely on them alone because there is a high chance of false readings due to colds, infections, and the like.

I was going to be on Coumadin to ensure that the port stayed clear, it thinned the blood slightly. I knew that my grandmother, who was on this drug, had to watch how much broccoli and grapefruit was in her diet. However, the oncologist said that I didn't have to worry about that because I was only going to be on a very low dose of 1 milligram.

He let me ask as many questions as I wanted, and he never lost his composure or rushed me. This behavior made me feel like he genuinely cared about what happened to me.

Once all the house-keeping was taken care of, I went to have my first chemotherapy treatment via the port. The nurses used ethyl chloride, a topical anesthetic that they called freezy spray, to chill the skin around my port. After that, they told me to take a deep breath and poked a needle into the port, and I didn't feel a thing. It was great!

In addition to Pepcid and Benadryl, the pre-chemotherapy cocktail included the following:

> Aranesp (darbepoetin alfa): a man-made form of a protein that helps your body to produce red blood cells. The amount of this natural protein may be reduced when you have kidney failure or use certain medications. Thus, Aranesp is used to treat anemia (a lack of red blood cells).

> Ativan (lorazepam), which is in a group of drugs called benzo-diazepines. It affects chemicals in the brain that may become unbalanced and cause anxiety. We wouldn't want any extra anxiety now, would we?

> Decadron (dexamethasone), which is used for treating certain conditions associated with decreased adrenal gland function.

Aloxi (palonosetron) blocks the actions of chemicals in the body that can trigger nausea and vomiting. It is used regularly to prevent these symptoms from being caused by medicine treating cancer (chemotherapy). This was the time-released anti-nausea medicine that the oncologist had mentioned.

Normal saline, which is 0.9 percent NaCl (sodium chloride or salt). This means that for every 100 milliliters of water, there are 0.9 grams of NaCl. This is equivalent to 9.0 grams per liter or 0.009 grams per milliliter. It is considered a sterile solution when delivered intravenously.

After administering these medicines, they proceeded with the first of the two chemotherapy drugs, Adriamycin (doxorubicin). It belongs to a group of medicines known as antitumor antibiotics and is used to treat some kinds of cancer. The drug sheet the oncologist gave me listed a slew of rare, occasional, and common side effects, one of which was the hair loss I knew was coming.

Part-way through the treatment, they pushed the second part of the treatment into the IV. It was a drug called Cytoxan (cyclophosphamide). It belongs to a group of medicines known as alkylating agents, which add an alkyl group to the DNA that interferes with DNA replication. It is used to treat some kinds of cancer. The drug sheet contained a whole list of possible side effects that could occur. It was all scary stuff!

The treatment was expected to take three to four hours, after all of the pre-medication was completed. After a little while, John went to the deli and brought back lunch. My normal order at the time was an Italian hero with Italian dressing and no onions. I just loved that sandwich. Come to think of it, I haven't had a craving for it since that year. Being stuck to the chair for many hours while the drugs were administered was very boring. We sat and watched television, and I fell asleep. I'm thinking that John did as well. When the treatment was finished, I again took a deep breath as they pulled the needle out of the port. It didn't hurt at all.

Two days later, I went back to the oncology department for a shot of Neulastin (a white blood cell booster). It burned when they injected it the first time, so they told me to make sure that in the future I ask them to push it slower to cause less discomfort The drug gave me body aches for a couple of days, but those were tolerable.

So, I had one treatment down, and only three more to go for this part of the protocol. On the Fridays between my treatment sessions, I went in for them to check my weight, platelets, red blood cells, white blood cells, and so forth to ensure that my body was handling everything okay and rebounding in a timely manner.

John took me to most of my chemotherapy appointments. I was not comfortable letting other people into my circle and see me as I had all of those chemicals going into my body. But there were two instances when he couldn't take me because of a work conflict, so my mom took me to one, and my aunt Maggie took me to the other. I want to thank each of them here for taking me to my treatments.

Despite all the research I had done, I was actually embarrassed and shy about my cancer treatment. I felt like it was my battle, and no one around me could or would really understand how I felt or what I was experiencing because they hadn't gone through it themselves (and I did not wish this experience on them). In case I ever came off as selfish or ungrateful, I want to apologize to my family now for any times that I might have been hard to live with. I love you all very much!

Chapter 13

The Aftereffects

Overall, I felt great the whole weekend after my first chemotherapy treatment. I thought, *If it keeps up like this, the process will be absolutely wonderful—it won't really impact my day-to-day life with my family.* I'm hoping that you can guess what eventually happened.

I took the girls to the local park that weekend, and we had a great time. My brother was surprised to see me out at the park because he knew people who needed to stay in bed following their chemo treatments. I told him that I felt good, so I was out and about, trying to keep my life as normal as possible.

Similar to the stories my brother heard, my friend with inflammatory breast cancer would end up sick and in bed for the whole week following her treatments. I kept my fingers crossed that the same thing wouldn't happen to me.

I went into the office on Monday and Tuesday that week, and then I worked from home on Wednesday, which was a good decision because I spent a lot of time in the bathroom. It was not a good day. Thursday, however, was a good day. There are good days and bad days, and you just have to roll with them as they come if you want to stay sane.

On the morning of March 5, I went to a post-operative appointment for the surgeon to check on my port. He said that everything looked great, and he was happy to hear that I was able to use it for my first chemotherapy treatment. The two ladies in the office there, both named Barbara, were amazing. One of them had had breast cancer and used the same doctors I was working with. She was doing well, and that gave me positive thoughts.

The same day, I went to get my between-treatment finger stick at the oncology office. My white blood cell count was very low a 1. I told him about a cough that I seemed to be getting, and he gave me a prescription for an antibiotic to help with the white blood cells, prevent infection, and so on. The doctor asked me to come back in five days to get my counts checked again.

I kept calling my hair salon that week to check on the status of the wig, but it was not in yet. I got really nervous, because the oncologist had said that I would start to lose my hair around the second treatment, which was only one week away.

Chapter 14

The Holistic Approach

On March 9, my mom took me to see a holistic doctor who was also a licensed chiropractor. I went in partially open-minded, especially because he helped so many of my family and friends. I had even sent a friend from work to see him when she felt like crap from taking so many osteoporosis medications starting in her early thirties. He got her off of that medicine, stopped her aches and pains, and helped her to regain bone mass and density. So I figured that I would give this treatment a whirl too.

The doctor was trained in Eastern medicines, and he used methods that didn't include blood tests, pain, or invasiveness. He had me hold a metal rod, attached to a machine, in my left hand. There was a piece of metal that looked like a plate with a wire attached to it. It led to another piece of metal, and he touched my right hand with it to make a complete circuit. This way he could listen to my body. He introduced a small vial, which looked like a fuse, into the circuit by placing it on the metal plate. By listening to the different tones from the machine, he could diagnose what was going on inside my body. He could also test different supplements and see if they would work for me by interpreting the different tones. This experience made me realize why you sometimes get sicker after taking a regularly prescribed medication and you go back to get a different prescription. It is because the particular drug didn't work with your body's machine. It's like putting diesel gas in an engine that only takes unleaded—it will ruin the engine or at least not allow it to run properly.

Well, the doctor discovered that my body was not producing sufficient white blood cells. There are three areas of your body that create white blood cells (the Lymph system, thymus, and spleen); two of those were not working. Therefore, my immune system was shot. This explained why I was constantly getting colds and every fall or winter I got bronchitis. He also said I had something in my body called the adenovirus. He said that nine out of ten people who come to him with a form of cancer have this virus. He told me that it had been in my system for a really long time, and at some point due to my low immune system, the virus compromised my cells and created a mutated cell, which led to the cancer. He said that once we got rid of the virus, there would be no more cancer in my future.

He recommended that since I was already diagnosed with cancer and had surgery, I should continue with my Western medicine protocols of chemotherapy and radiation. He would work with me to help counteract how the treatments would affect the rest of my body.

During this first visit, he worked on elevating my white blood cell count and clearing my lymphatic system and thymus via supplements and laser acupuncture. The beeping sounds were strange yet interesting. He explained things as he went along so that I understood how he knew what my body needed.

I mentioned that I had been drinking Mylanta on and off for a long time and I had moved on to Zantac to calm my burning stomach. As soon as I mentioned this, he put a vial into the circuit, and when he touched my hand, the machine made a different kind of noise. He said that I had H. pylori in my stomach, which causes ulcers and related symptoms.

Based on my initial consultation, he started me on a homeopathic regimen that included the following items.

o   A supplement to rid my body of the adenovirus that we feel caused my cancer.
o   Lime water to reduce the amount of acid in my body, as acid breeds viruses, cancer, and other illnesses. Your body needs to have a pH balance that is more alkaline than acidic because diseases breed in an acidic environment.

o   A supplement to treat the H. pylori bacteria.

o   Crotalus combo #B and #C, antiviral supplements.

o   Monolaurin, another antiviral supplement.

o   MGN3, an immune builder.

o   T-Cell, an immune builder for the thymus.

o   Lymphomyosot, an immune builder to clean out and rebuild the lymph system.

o   Bio C Plus, an immune builder to detoxify and rebuild the lymph system.

o   Sublingual B12, a red blood cell booster.

The holistic doctor also had me start drinking a quarter cup of pure aloe vera water first thing every morning to help heal my stomach, and in less than a month, I no longer need to take the over-the-counter medicines for ulcer relief. When I saw the oncologist, I mentioned the H. pylori. He knew what it was, so I felt even more confident with my choice to venture into alternative medicine as part of my treatment.

C h a p t e r   1 5

The Treatments Continue

I went back to see the oncologist on March 10, and my white blood cell count was up to 9.5, which was just inside the upper limits of the accepted guidelines. At my weigh-in, I was down three pounds from the one on February 27. I was thrilled. The people in the lab said that I should not be trying to lose weight right now. I smiled and nodded to make them think that I was acknowledging what they were saying, but I said to myself, "*If I want to lose weight, then I will!*"

I reviewed my tests with the oncologist, and he said the results of the bone scan and CAT scan were both good. In other words, there was no sign of cancer in my organs or bones. Yippee! I also picked up the letter to the airline, and I felt sad and disappointed all over again when I held it. I provided him with a list of the holistic supplements that I was planning on taking. He looked at the list and said they were okay for me to take, but he asked me not to take them the day before, day of, or day after treatment, just like the conventional vitamins. I asked him about massage therapy, and he said that was fine. Someone had told me that it helped work the chemicals out of your body. I asked about the ciprofloxacin I was on, and he told me to stop taking that.

At this point, I decided to start tracking my blood work. I was a Microsoft Excel enthusiast, so each week I brought home my CBC blood checks and put them in a spreadsheet. It was color coded, and I often asked my oncologist about why certain markers were always low while others were always high. I came up with a nick-name for myself: the oncologist's little PITA (pain in the a———). I drove him nuts at every visit, but it made me feel better to take an active role in my treatment and see how my body was handling it.

Definition	Weight	Normal Range	2/20/2004 173.00	2/27/2004 175.00	3/5/2004	3/10/2004 172.00	3/12/2004 171.00	3/19/2004	3/22/2004	3/26/2004 169.00	4/2/2004	4/5/2004	4/9/2004 171.00	4/16/2004
WBC	x10^3/µl	4.6 - 10.2	4.3	5.1	1	9.5	7.5	2.4	5.3	13.8	2.7	2.9	7.7	2.6
RBC	x10^6/µl	4.04 - 5.48	4.28	3.93	3.54	3.76	3.86	3.46	3.24	3.26	3.2	2.78	3.17	2.89
HGB	g/dL	12.2 - 16.2	13.9	12.7	11.7	12.3	12.5	11.4	10.7	10.6	10.3	9.1	10.4	9.6
HCT	%	37.7 - 47.9	40.5	37.3	32.8	35	36.6	31.7	30.1	30.1	29.5	25.2	30.1	26.6
MCV	fL	80 - 97	94.6	95	92.7	93.2	94.8	91.6	92.8	92.2	92.2	90.6	94.8	92.2
MCH	pg	27.0 - 31.2	32.5	32.3	33.1	32.7	32.4	32.9	33	32.5	32.2	32.7	32.8	33.2
MCHC	g/dL	31.8 - 35.4	34.3	34	35.7	35.1	34.7	36	35.5	35.2	34.9	36.1	34.6	36.1
RDW	%	11.6 - 14.8	13.1	13.4	12.4	13.2	12.9	13.5	12.5	12.7	13.4	13.8	14.5	15.4
PLT	x10^3/µl	142 - 424	230	231	122	223	332	273	198	213	292	169	275	227
MPV	fL	7.4 - 10.4	9.3	9.2	9.2	9.9	8.9	9	9.4	9.1	8.1	8.5	9.6	8.1
LYMPH	%	10 - 50	38.2 R2	33.7	51.4	25.8 R2	21.4	20.5	23.3 R2	14.7 R2	17.2	28.3 R2	15.7 R2	21.5
MID	%		9.5	17.4	6.1	6.4	5.5	7.7 R2	13.3	5.6	7.5	9.4	5.8	5.3
GRAN	%	37 - 80	52.3 R3	48.9 RM2	41.5 R4	67.8	73.1	71.8 R4	63.4 R3	79.7	75.3	62.3	78.5	73.2
LYNPH	x10^3/µl	0.6 - 3.4	1.6 R2	1.7	0.5	2.5 R2	1.6	0.5	1.2 R2	2.0 R2	0.5	0.8 R2	1.2 R2	0.6
MID	x10^3/µl		0.4	0.9	0.1	0.6	0.4	0.2 R2	0.7	0.8	0.2	0.3	0.4	0.1
GRAN	x10^3/µl	2.0 - 6.9	2.2 R3	2.5 RM	0.4 R4	6.4	5.5	1.7 R4	3.4 R3	11	2	1.8	6	1.9

Higher than average

Lower than average

Chemo dates

CBC Tracking

4/21/2004	4/23/2004	4/30/2004	5/7/2004	5/14/2004	5/21/2004	5/28/2004	6/4/2004	6/7/2004	6/11/2004	6/18/2004	6/21/2004	6/25/2004	7/6/2004	8/17/2004	8/23/2004
169.00	170.00	167.00	167.50		166.80	166.00	166.00	167.00		165.00	166.00	165.00	168.00		
6.8	7	4	1.8	3.7	3.8	2.6	4.5	7.5	7.9	6.5	9.5	10.9	10.8	3.1	3.1
2.85	2.71	2.99	3.04	3.42	3.81	3.75	3.94	3.71	3.92	3.65	3.56	3.74	3.46	3.51	3.58
9.4	8.8	10.2	10	11.6	12.9	12.4	13.4	12.1	13.4	12.1	12.1	12.2	11.3	11.4	11.6
27	26.2	29.8	30	33.4	37.4	36.2	38.4	36.4	37.9	35.2	34.6	35.5	33.6	32.7	34
94.8	96.6	99.8	98.6	97.8	98.2	96.6	97.4	98.2	96.7	96.5	97.1	95	97.1	93.1	94.9
33	32.5	34.1	32.9	33.9	33.9	33.1	34	32.6	34.2	33.2	34	32.6	32.7	32.5	32.4
34.8	33.6	34.2	33.3	34.7	34.5	34.3	34.9	33.2	35.4	34.4	35	34.4	33.6	34.9	34.1
14.4	15	20.2	21.4	19.8	18.8	17.3	16.4	16.7	15.7	15.8	15.4	15.6	15.9	16.6	15.3
129	197	304	198	235	187	183	163	171	184	184	269	192	200	265	175
9.6	9	8.8	8.4	2.9	9.2	8.9	9.1	8.6	9.6	9.5	9.8	9.7	8.7	8.2	8.4
19.2 R2	20.4 R2	17.0 R2	70.7	59.1	43.5	60.1	40.9	12.1	15.4 R2	24.3	12.3	10.4	9.7	31.6 R2	34.5 R2
6.4		8.8	7.7	11.5	6.3	4.6	7.4	7.6 R2	24.7 R2	8.5 R3	4.2	6.0 R2	3.4	6.8	12.9
74.4	74.2	74.2	21.6 R4	29.4 RM	50.2	35.3	51.7 R3	80.3 R3	59.9 8M	67.2 RM	83.5	83.6	86.9	61.6	52.6 RM
1.3 R2		0.7 R2	1.3	2.2	1.7	1.6	1.8	0.9	1.2 R2	1.6	1.2	1.1	1	1.0 R2	1.1 R2
0.4		0.4	0.1	0.4	0.2	0.1	0.3	0.6 R2	2.0 R2	0.6 R3	0.4	0.7 R2	0.4	0.2	0.4
5.1		3	0.4 R4	1.1 RM	1.9	0.9	2.3 R3	6.1 R3	4.7 RM	4.4 RM	7.9	9.1	9.4	1.9	1.6 RM

On March 10, I submitted the necessary paperwork to the airline to begin processing the refund for the tickets. It was a very sad day, as if flags flew at half-mast.

On Friday, March 12, I again worked from home for a few hours before my treatment. I complained to the oncologist about a headache and mentioned my frustrations with bathroom issues and feeling like crap. He offered me information on a support group, but I declined it. I was not one to share with others, and I did not want to subject myself to their negative stories.

I had lost another pound in two days' time. I agree that it's not the healthiest way to lose weight, but I'm open to whatever works. On the plus side, my white blood cell count was perfect. My second treatment consisted of the same regimen of three or four hours as the first one. I got my Italian sandwich, watched some television, and took a nap. Now I had two treatments down, two to go! I went home and worked for a few more hours that evening to keep my mind busy. I couldn't just sit around.

On March 14, I went back for my shot of Neulastin. I remembered what I had learned from my first injection and I asked the nurse to administer it more slowly. It went a little better, but my body still ached for a few days. I stayed positive, thinking that these side effects were a small price to pay for a full life with my family.

I stayed in bed for half of the weekend after the second treatment and was now really glad that I had opted for Friday appointments. I didn't want to miss work if at all possible. My parents came over to watch the girls so that John could go grocery shopping. They folded the laundry too. I felt weak and embarrassed and so many other emotions. I could hear them laughing and having a great time while I was lying in bed, feeling miserable. I wanted to be out there, but I just couldn't muster the energy. I knew they were helping me because they loved me. My family was and still is the best support group ever.

I decided to do some research on the drugs in my protocol. I'm glad I didn't do the research prior to starting the treatment, because I'm not sure that I would have chosen to do it. Some of the things I learned where heart stoppers, but please don't let this scare you. I simply want to mention it as part of my journey.

I went to work on March 15 and 16. I realized that I got very tired in the afternoon, so I arranged it that I would leave the office around 2:30 p.m. and drive home. I would then work from home the rest of the afternoon, this way I wasn't sitting in traffic while I was so exhausted.

By March 16, I started to feel postnasal drip, congestion, and a cough. I thought, *This is absolutely ridiculous. I can't catch a break!*

I worked from home on Wednesday, March 17. Wednesdays became the day I called my "issues" day where I spent an awful lot of time in the bathroom with little notice, so I worked from home on Wednesdays for the foreseeable future. It was nice and quiet there with Emma in day care and Megan in school all day.

Chapter 16

Family Support

About this time, my dad started coming over every morning to help with my daughters, as John had to be at work before the girls were up. Megan was five years old at the time. She had been born at twenty-eight weeks and spent a month in the neonatal intensive care unit. As mentioned previously, she has mild cerebral palsy. She started receiving physical therapy services from the time she was about fourteen months old. Megan didn't walk until after she was two years old, with the help of a walker and braces on both of her legs. She wore her braces to school every day, but all of the other children were so accepting of her.

My dad would stretch out her muscles every morning before putting on her braces and getting her on to the bus. My dad also took Emma to day care every day. He didn't want me to be near the dozens of children who could be carrying different kinds of viruses. My dad was amazing! What's more, my whole family was amazing through this whole journey.

Megan ready for school and waiting for the bus:

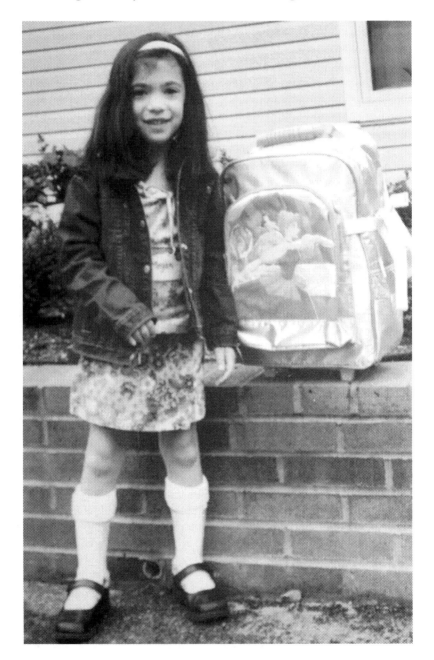

Chapter 17

Eastern plus Western Medicine

On March 17, I went back to the natural health-care provider, and he used the same machine to listen to all of the different sounds my body generated. Then he used laser acupuncture to work on my digestive system, as it was not reacting to the chemotherapy very well.

I worked from my office on March 18 and 19, but I tried to keep to myself because my immune system was not in the best of shape and my susceptibility to illnesses was heightened because of my low white blood cell count. Offices are not quite as bad as day care centers in regard to germs, but they are not far off.

On Friday, March 19, I went to my appointment for blood work between chemotherapy sessions, and my white blood cell and red blood cell counts were both low again. I declined an additional shot of Neulastin and told them I was working on this holistically. They were not happy with me, and one nurse said, "I will have to note your chart that you refused the injection."

I replied, "Well, go ahead then." I wanted to say, "Really? It's up to me how I want to handle my treatment. It's my life." But I didn't. The PITA was at it again. They asked me to come back in on the following Monday to check my blood counts again.

I visited my holistic provider on March 20, and he worked on rebalancing my immune system and thymus gland as well as my blood cells. He performed laser acupuncture and gave me some Sublingual B12 (a booster supplement for red blood cells) to help get my numbers back within the oncologist's guidelines. He also explained that my counts were fine, for me. It was just that my numbers did not fit into their standard ranges. I always knew that I was special, and now this was proof that I'm not like everybody else.

On Monday, March 22, I went back to the oncology office so that they could check my blood cell counts. My white blood cell count was finally in line, but I had a cough, nasal congestion, and pink eye. They prescribed a topical ointment for my eye, but that was it. So I didn't need that extra shot of Neulastin after all. I wanted to stick my tongue out and give the chemotherapy nurse a great big raspberry, but that wouldn't have been very nice, would it?

Shortly after my second treatment, my hair started falling out as predicted. I called Sal, who said that the wig had finally come in but was totally unshaped. He spent many hours cutting the hair on the wig to get it all shaped up for me. I worked from home that week—no hair and no wig meant I was not going in to the office. I called my boss and explained what was going on, and he totally understood. He said that he knew what a hard worker I was, and he had no concerns about my ability to get my job done regardless of my location.

Megan tried to understand when I explained that the medicine I was taking was going to make my hair fall out, but at five years old, I'm not sure how she could have known what I meant. At first, my hair came out a few strands at a time, and then it started coming out in clumps. There are caps you can wear to catch the hair while you sleep, but they were not comfortable at all, so I slept with a towel over my pillow to prevent making a mess. Soon, my head became very uncomfortable, and the patches of missing hair looked very ugly. I felt that I looked like a Holocaust victim, even though I could never truly know what that experience was like. I trimmed my hair as short as possible, but it didn't fully help. When the stubble rubbed on the handkerchief I wore to cover my head, it really hurt. When the girls were taking a nap one day, I went into the bathroom, looked in the mirror, and told myself that if I was going to lose my hair, then I wanted to be the one to make it happen. I took John's razor and shaved my head, and I immediately felt so much more comfortable. When Megan got up from her nap, she took one look at my head and asked, "What happened to your hair,

Mommy?" I asked her if she remembered what I told her about the medicine I was taking. She shrugged her shoulders gently and then rubbed and kissed my head.

As I had for the past couple of treatments, I worked on the morning of Friday, March 26, and then went to the oncologist for my third treatment. At my weigh-in I had lost two more pounds during the last two weeks. Then they did the finger stick, and my white blood cell count was higher than the upper limit. I complained about my ongoing cough and nasal congestion, but this was not getting me anywhere, as you can see. I went into the treatment room and got all set up with my freezy spray and my pre-chemo cocktail. I cuddled up with my quilt and settled in for a long winters' nap. Oh, wait! That's the wrong story, but it really is boring sitting there for three or four hours. At the end of that appointment, I was glad that I could say, "Okay! Three treatments down, only one more to go!" I could finally see the light at the end of this tunnel, but I was still unsure what the next one would bring me. I also felt some concern because my body was not reacting very well to the first round of chemotherapy.

Two days later, I went in for my regular Neulastin shot. This visit was quick, and there was nothing exciting to report. I had the normal burning and body aches for a few days after.

I spent almost the entire weekend in bed. I was ready to stop treatment. I was miserable, but I thought about my girls and the future. I kept running all of the different scenarios through my head. What would happen if I stopped all treatment, if I continued both the regular and holistic treatments, or if I decided to just go the holistic route? Would the girls be okay if something happened to me? If I stopped my treatment plan, did it mean I was giving up and possibly letting cancer win? Did I really still have cancer if they removed it in the surgery? This is such a hard decision for anyone to make. You don't ever want to be in those shoes. My husband wasn't on board with me quitting. I finally decided I was going to continue with my treatment because there were way too many unknowns. If I did decide to stop the treatment and something went wrong, I'd be doing the same what-if's but in the opposite direction, like what if I didn't stop the treatment? This was just way too much mental stress for me, which is not good for anyone, especially me.

The Hair, Part II

I was finally going to get my wig, and it was just in time for my sister's wedding. Sal brought it to my house on Sunday morning, March 28. I had known him for a long time, and I still felt strange around him without any hair but safe at the same time.

He spent a couple of hours shaping and styling the wig so that it looked natural on me. It felt weird. When I looked in the mirror, my reflection looked like me with a new do, but it didn't feel like that on my scalp. Overall, I was happy with the results.

I thanked Sal for all he had done for me, and he said to make sure that I came into the salon to get my hair done for my sister's wedding.

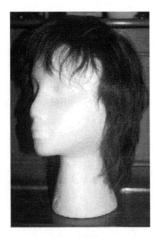

My Wig

As soon as I had my wig, I went back to working at the office from 8:00 a.m. to 2:30 p.m. every day but Wednesday, as mentioned in an earlier chapter. Work was the only constant in my life that helped me get through all of this other crap! I felt like I was in control of something, and my projects kept my mind busy. I am thankful every day that the company I worked for was willing and able to be flexible during this hard time in my life.

Chapter 19

The Low Whites

On March 29, I went to see the holistic practitioner, and he said that my white blood cells were low again, so he worked on that as well as my thymus and lymph system. He gave me more Sublingual B12 and Monolaurin (a homeopathic antibiotic) to help with the upper respiratory issues that I was experiencing as a result of the chemotherapy. I figured that the latter was worth trying, considering the oncologist wasn't helping much with this recurring issue.

Friday, April 2, was my next non-treatment week blood check. My white blood cell count was low again. For some reason I wasn't rebounding as fast as I should have been. I again complained about my cough and runny nose. When I lay down, it felt almost like I was trying to breathe liquid. I'd have to compare it to what it might feel like if you were drowning. I did not get much sleep when this happened, and the symptoms were more severe after each chemotherapy treatment. It was scary. When I told the oncologist that I was exhausted and needed to get some sleep before my sister's wedding the next day, he gave me a prescription for hydrocodone syrup and asked me to come back in on Monday to have my blood counts rechecked. I was getting pretty tired of these recurring rechecks by now.

Chapter 20

The Wedding

I was really nervous about going to my sister's wedding. There were going to be a lot of family and friends who knew me but hadn't seen me in a while. And now they were going to see me in this state. I wanted to be there for my sister, but at the same time, I wanted to stay in my secluded little world at home.

I took the super cough medicine Friday evening, and when I woke up on Saturday, April 3, I felt a little better. I had actually gotten some sleep. I got ready and headed over to the salon. I went in there like I had regular hair and got it washed and styled. The wig—or should I say my hair—looked very pretty when Sal was finished with it.

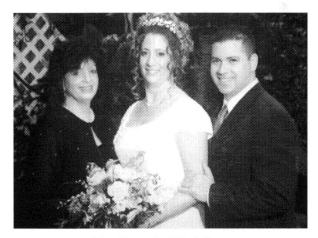

My Sister's Wedding

I had a nice time at the wedding, but I was a little tired. I got a lot of compliments on my whole ensemble. When I looked in the mirror back then, the wig looked to me like I had straightened my naturally wavy hair. Although when I look back at the pictures now, I can tell that it was a wig.

In fact, that's one new talent that I learned through my experience: I can usually tell when someone is wearing a wig. It is very hard to explain, but if you are reading this and you have ever been in the same situation, you will probably understand what I mean. For those of you who are unsure, I'm not going to give away the secrets for how you can tell because I don't think it's fair to those who are wearing wigs.

Chapter 21

Easter

On April 5, I went back to the oncology office for blood work, and my white blood cell count was still low. He wanted me to have an additional shot of Neulastin, but I declined. I proceeded to have a major discussion with my oncologist to understand why I was doing all of this, especially if they removed all of the cancer in the surgery. To me, that implied the drugs they were giving me were actually attacking my good cells. Somehow—I don't recall exactly how—he convinced me to continue.

From there, I went to see the holistic practitioner. He checked all the dosages of my supplements using the machine and adjusted my blood boosters. Then he used laser acupuncture to work on rebuilding my spleen and raising my white blood cell count.

The morning of April 9, I worked from home and then went to the oncologist. I found out that I had gained two pounds during the past two weeks. I was a little disappointed but planned to work on it for the next visit. My white blood cell counts were fine when I had my finger stick. The doctors got very worried between treatments, but the holistic treatments helped my body rebuild naturally over time rather than using extra chemicals, such as Neulastin injections. I had my fourth treatment, which concluded the first portion of my chemotherapy protocol. I took some paperwork with me to the infusion room so that I could keep up with my work. I also took a little nap. I was so glad that this phase of the treatment was finally coming to an end.

Two days later was Easter Sunday, April 11. As you might recall, the only good weekend I had after a treatment was the first one, way back in February, which now felt like a life-time ago. This time, I felt like death warmed over. I was pale, weak, tired, and cold. I just wanted to crawl into bed and veg out, but I went to my grandma's for Easter Dinner anyway. It was definitely not one of my good days. I was very self-conscious, and I didn't like the idea of my aunts, uncles, parents, cousins and grandmother seeing me in this condition. Everyone was great, but I could see the concern in their eyes. It was especially hard because they had all seen me looking so much more alive the week before at my sister's wedding.

On April 12, a Monday appointment because of the holiday, I went to the oncologist's office for my last Neulastin shot. The nurses listened to me and pushed the liquid slowly so that my arm didn't burn. I still had body aches for a few days after the shot, but since this was the last one, I was okay with it.

That afternoon, I had an appointment with my holistic practitioner, and he worked on my spleen and white blood cell counts to try to get a head start on the downward spirals that I usually had after chemo treatments.

Chapter 22

Emma's First Birthday Party

Emma's first birthday was on April 14, and we had the party on Sunday, April 18. In our family, we always have really big parties for first birthdays. Because we knew that I would be in the middle of treatment, we decided to have Emma's party at a local restaurant instead of at our house. We scheduled it for a non-treatment weekend, so the plan was for me to be feeling well.

Everyone had a really good time. Emma was very happy, and I felt really good. I had more color in my face and looked more alive than I had recently. I think that helped my family feel more comfortable about everything that I was going through. I am sure that it was very hard for my family to see me go through so many ups and downs, and they did a really good job of hiding their fears and only showing me their most supportive side.

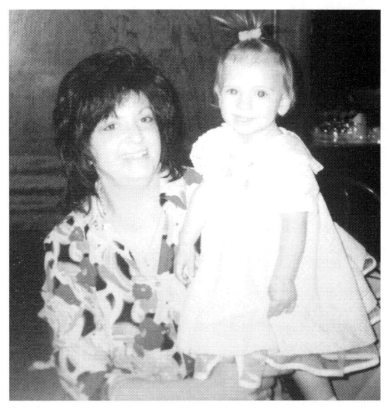

Emma's First Birthday

Chapter 23

Popping the Top

On a lighter note, the wig made my head really itchy. As soon as I walked in the door, I would rip the wig off and scratch my head like crazy. For some reason, we started calling this "popping my top." Megan thought this was hysterical. Then I put the wig on the Styrofoam head in the bathroom until I needed it the next day. She would ask, "Mom, are you going to pop your top?" We laughed about this over and over again!

I was so comfortable walking around with my bald head at home, but even so, there is not one picture of me with my bald head. I remember that I didn't want to have any photographs that immortalized this time in my life.

I was so used to being wig-free at home. One day, John, Megan, Emma, and I were leaving for the mall, and we had walked out of the house, locked the front door, and started to go down the front steps when Megan shouted, "Mom, you forgot your hair!" I stopped in my tracks and touched the top of my head. She was right! I had gone out of the house without my hair. I unlocked the door quickly, ran inside, put my wig on, and then we went off to the mall. We had a great big laugh about that.

Chapter 24

The Taxotere Protocol Begins

On April 16, I went to the oncologist for my blood-count check, and as usual, my white blood cell count was low. They started me on a new drug, Aranesp. It would prepare me for the second set of chemotherapy by combatting the effects that the Taxotere could have on the red blood cell counts, potentially leading to anemia (fatigue). As long as my blood counts rebounded, I would start the Taxotere protocol on April 23. The oncologist wanted me to come back for testing on Wednesday because he was afraid that my body would not be ready for treatment on the following Friday.

I was continuing to see my holistic practitioner regularly, so I went to see him on the afternoon of April 16. He worked on my spleen, thymus, and lymph system as well as working on balancing my pH levels. I also continued to take Monolaurin to treat my respiratory issues. They had not totally cleared up, but they were definitely improving.

On Wednesday, April 21, when I went back to the oncologist, my white blood cell levels were good. It seemed that the holistic treatment and time had helped again. Oh, I almost forgot to mention that I lost the two pounds I had gained at my last weigh-in. This made me feel like I had accomplished a goal and I was actually in control of something.

On Friday, April 23, I was about to start down the path of my next chemotherapy adventure: Taxotere! If you remember, the oncologist and I had agreed to a calendar of four weeks on, one week off for the Taxotere treatment, for a total of fourteen weeks.

My white blood cell count was fine, but when I had my weigh-in, I had gained a pound back in two days. I chalked it up to water weight and moved on. The oncologist explained that this part of the treatment had a lower risk of impacting my white blood cell counts, so I no longer needed the Neulastin shots. Thank goodness there would be no more burning arm and body aches! On the other hand, there was a much greater chance of Taxotere negatively impacting my red blood cell counts, so fatigue could be more prevalent. There are ups and downs on this journey, like a roller coaster that you don't want to be on but you can't get off.

My first Taxotere treatment began with the same lovely freezy spray followed by the same pre-chemotherapy mix I had with the Cytoxan and Adriamycin protocol: Aloxi, Decadron, Ativan, and Aranesp in a normal saline solution. After these drugs were infused, the Taxotere was also administered via the port.

When I woke up on Sunday, April 25, I thought I had the worst intestinal virus in history. I spent an awful lot of time in the bathroom. I really thought that my insides were going to end up on my outsides.

I went to see my holistic practitioner the next day, and he treated me for the same low blood cell count issues as usual. I told him about my awful weekend and the twenty-four-hour bug that I had. He tested me for viruses, and all of the beeping sounds were normal. He said that how I felt had nothing to do with a virus and everything to do with the side effects from the new chemotherapy treatment. He added iron to my list of supplements to help me rebuild myself, as my body had lost a lot of nutrients over the past day.

I went to the oncologist on April 30 to have my second Taxotere treatment. My weigh-in went wonderfully: I had lost three pounds in one week. It was probably because I was so sick, but I didn't care about that at the moment. My white blood cell levels were fine, so I was able to have my second treatment. I told the doctor that my fingertips were starting to ache and felt very sensitive. I also told him that I had finished the prescription for my upper respiratory issues, but my chest was still congested. I told him about the virus that I had the prior weekend, and he noted in my file that I complained about "mild nausea and loose stools." Then he included Pepcid in my pre-chemotherapy cocktail and gave me Anzemet (an anti-nausea medication) to help with the symptoms I told him about.

Two days later, I ended up with the same symptoms that I had the prior weekend. The Pepcid did not help at all. This was just great! It really was not a virus. I couldn't imagine repeating this process for twelve more treatments. Could you?

On May 3, I called the doctor and said that I experienced vomiting and diarrhea two days after each of my Taxotere treatments. They told me to stop taking the Anzemet, as it had the potential side effect of causing diarrhea. All of these drugs are supposed to fix one thing, but they have all of these other potential side effects.

I went to see my holistic practitioner, and he did a balancing to tweak the dosage of the supplements I was taking and prescribed a new supplement to detox my liver. We were trying to help my body have less of an acute reaction to the Taxotere.

I went to have my third Taxotere treatment on May 7. My weight was up a half a pound, but I was still down a net two and a half pounds, so I wasn't worried. But my white blood cell count was way too low (1.8, when the minimum guideline was 4.6). They were a bit worried, so they also checked my temperature. A body temperature of a hundred degrees was an early warning sign that an infection was brewing. I did not have a fever, but my third treatment was postponed due to my low white blood cell count. They gave me a shot of Neupogen to help with the blood count recovery and fight infection.

My body was in a shambles. The Taxotere was wreaking havoc on my organs, and I needed some help. I went to see my holistic practitioner on May 10, where I had my spleen, liver, and lymph systems cleared and my white blood cells boosted via laser acupuncture. He also adjusted my supplement dosage. Since my treatment was pushed back, I now had the next week to relax and recuperate.

Chapter 25

The Thank-You

During that week, I finally had some time to sit down and write one big well-deserved thank-you note to all of the people who helped me and those who donated to the wig fund that my aunt Santa had started earlier in the year. I was and still am so grateful to have such wonderful, supportive, and caring family and friends.

So many people wanted to help in any and every way they could. They offered everything from time and money to a shoulder to cry on or an ear to listen. I was humbled by the outpouring of generosity. It was a great feeling to experience all of this love, and you should not wait for tragedy to strike to show someone how important he or she is to you.

May 11, 2004

Dear; Mom and Dad, Christine and Brian, Vinny and Jennifer, Mom, Grandma, Aunt Santa, Aunt Angie and Uncle Steve, Sabrina, Anthony, Alicia and Joe, Deniece and Louis, Aunt Maggie and Uncle Jim, Uncle Ron, Charlie and Jennifer, Andrea and Frank, Berica and Brandon, Gen and Richie, Betty and Lenny, Steve and Danielle, Julie, and Maryann,

When Aunt Santa told me that everyone who cared about me wanted to do "something" to help, I told her that it wasn't necessary. But she still wanted to do something, so she came up with the idea of a "wig fund", since my health insurance covers everything except for a wig......which makes no sense to me, but what are you going to do.

I just wanted to thank all of you for your thoughtfulness and your generous contributions to the "wig fund".

I worked with my hairdresser who has been doing my hair for 21 years now, and he hooked me up with the "best". I now have my "hair". It is made with real hair, and I can wash it and blow-dry it (although not every day). It's longer than my usual style, but everyone says that if you didn't know my old hair, you wouldn't know this was a wig.

My hairdresser left it long so that we could have "fun" with it. So next month if I want to get a haircut, or get it highlighted, I can do whatever I want to it.

All of the contributions collected, were not spent on this wig. I was informed that I will need a second wig that has holes in it, when my hair starts to grow in. So I have put the remainder of the "wig fund" in the bank and will use it to purchase the second wig later on this year.

I also wanted to take a moment to thank Christine, Brian, Vin and Jen for their thoughtfulness and generosity during this difficult time. For those not aware, they have been having my house cleaned every other week while all of this is going on. They tried to talk me into it when I was pregnant with Emma and I said no thanks, I'll clean my own house. So this time they didn't ask me, they just told me that they were doing it. It is absolutely wonderful! Now that Emma's all over the place, it really helps having the floors cleaned and I really haven't had the energy to do it.

All is going well for the most part. Everyone's been chipping in and helping out when I have my "not so good" days.

I am very fortunate to have the most wonderful family and friends around and I thank you over and over for being so wonderful and being there for my family and me.

Thank you very much!!

Love,

Joanne

Thank You Note

Chapter 26

Treatment Postponed

On May 14, one week later, I went back to try to have my third Taxotere treatment, and although my white blood cell count was definitely improved, it was only 3.7, which was still too low for a treatment. I refused an additional Neupogen injection, but they gave me a shot of Aranesp to help treat my anemia. The delay actually worked in my favor this time, because I had already planned to skip this week for treatment to attend a birthday party. I cannot remember who it was for, but it must have been important because I noted that I had cleared it with the oncologist ahead of time.

I went to the holistic practitioner on Monday, May 17, and he worked on building up my thymus, spleen, bone marrow, and lymph system. He performed laser acupuncture and gave me a white blood cell booster. We were trying to get my body to snap back so that I could continue treatments.

I had my next weigh-in and blood cell count on May 21. The good news was that I had lost another pound, but my white blood cell count was still low at 3.8. They looked at the rest of the blood work and said that since my HCT, MCV, LYMPH, and GRAN markers had improved, I could actually have my third Taxotere treatment. The oncologist was also concerned that if I took too many weeks off in a row, it could impact the overall effectiveness of the treatment. Even though they gave me Pepcid, I again experienced diarrhea and vomiting.

My fingernails became even more sensitive than they already were. Have you ever caught the edges of your fingernails on something (like a car door or the edge of a counter) and bent them back slightly? My fingertips and nails felt like that all of the time. It was very uncomfortable. On the plus side, I was thankful that my fingernails didn't actually fall off. You must keep finding the glass-half-full perspective whenever possible, because there are plenty of times when the glass can feel empty and bone dry.

On May 24, my holistic practitioner and I worked on my nutrition. We needed to do something different. What we had been doing was helping, but it wasn't helping enough. So, we decided to start me on vitamin C and not tell the oncologist. He checked my bone marrow, spleen, thymus, and lymph system and also adjusted my acidity, iron levels, and adrenals with some B5 and B6.

I went to the oncologist for my fourth Taxotere treatment on May 28. My white and red blood cell counts were both too low, so I couldn't go through with the treatment that day. I declined the Neupogen injection. They wanted me to come back in three days to check my blood cell counts, but I refused. I was getting sick of the testing and waiting and not having high enough blood cell counts. I told them that I wasn't coming back in until June 4 for my normal appointment and left the office. I had lost another pound, but that did not help my mood this time.

Chapter 27

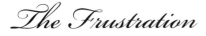
The Frustration

I was starting to get very frustrated. It had been six weeks since I had officially started the Taxotere protocol, and I had only gotten three treatments. I should have been on my fifth one by now. I thought, *There is no way I can continue with this timeline!*

You see, I had a timeline mapped out in my head based on my initial visit to the oncologist, and my goal was to be done with both the chemotherapy and radiation treatments by Labor Day 2004. And because I am such a control freak, I needed to stay on that schedule no matter what. It allowed me to see the light at the end of the tunnel, the finish line. Without that end in sight, I was seriously having a hard time making myself continue the treatments. My husband saw how miserable I was and that it was impacting our lives terribly. So, we decided that we would meet with the oncologist to talk about this. In my mind, I had already decided that when I went to my next appointment, I was going to tell the oncologist that I was done.

At my appointment on June 4, there was no weight change, and my white blood cell count was 4.5 (just under the lower limit of 4.6). This meant no treatment again. This really upset me. John and I had a very long conversation with the oncologist. We reviewed all of my treatments, the side effects, and my body's reactions. I told the doctor that I was leaning toward not continuing chemotherapy treatment. He was very concerned and repeated that he treats all of his patients like he would his wife or daughter, and he'd be terribly worried if they didn't continue. That applied to me as well. I told him that physically and mentally, I could no longer handle the way the treatments were going, and I didn't want the weekly Taxotere treatments anymore. I said that I was contemplating alternative medicine, and I was very concerned about the possibility of secondary cancers as a result of the chemotherapy.

Gaining steam, I asked why I needed to proceed with radiation treatments. If doses of radiation aren't good for healthy people, why was it good for me? He said that the chemotherapy drugs (I called them poison) that they put in my body would not reach the actual tumor site because of scar tissue from the surgery. It treats the whole body and works to attack and kill any radical cancer cells that might be floating around.

In contrast, the radiation treats the actual tumor site and the surrounding scar tissue. I begrudgingly agreed to the radiation treatments and asked when I would be able to actually start them. The oncologist said I could begin within two weeks after my last chemotherapy treatment, when the blood cell counts should have bounced back. My friend had told me that at least three appointments were necessary to get you ready before the actual treatments started, so I asked if I could start making appointments with the radiation group. I still wanted to move things along as quickly as possible.

By the end of the visit, we came up with a compromise. If you remember, there were two possible options regarding the timing of the Taxotere treatments: four bulk treatments over eight weeks, or twelve mini treatments over fourteen weeks. We had initially gone with the latter. Due to my reactions, I had only had three mini treatments so far, which was the equivalent to one bulk treatment. We decided to switch over to the bulk treatments. I told the oncologist that I would only commit to doing one bulk treatment and then I would see how my body responded before proceeding any further. Even though he did not agree, he understood and did not push me.

He also prescribed an oral anti-nausea medication I could take at home called Zofran. It was amazing and really took the edge off the queasiness. I mentioned this medicine to my friend dealing with inflammatory breast cancer, as she was having major nausea issues as well. However, the treatment center she was going to said that although it was available, they could not prescribe it for her because it was manufactured by a drug family that did not belong to their cancer treatment group. How ridiculous is that!

Chapter 28

The Light at the End of the Chemotherapy Tunnel

On June 7, a Monday, I weighed in and had my blood cell count checked. I was up a pound, but after everything else I had been going through, that was the least of my worries. My white blood cell count was right in the middle of the acceptable range—perfect.

Before my treatment, I had another long discussion with the oncologist. I mentioned that the soles of my feet were peeling, and I was seeing changes in my nails. We again discussed the benefits of continuing, and I restated that at this point I was only agreeing to that day's Taxotere treatment. He amended the treatment plan in my file to show that I was switching to the bulk version, and then I went and had my treatment.

I wasn't enjoying this anymore. Oh who was I kidding, I was never enjoying it. It was definitely getting harder to keep my chin up and trudge along. Now that I had finished what equated to my second bulk treatment, there were only two left. I realized that if I continued with this regimen, I would meet my Labor Day deadline after all.

I also saw the holistic practitioner that day for a quick check, and there were no adjustments needed. He told me to keep taking my supplements, and we talked about how the chemotherapy treatments were affecting my body. He took the time to listen and reassured me that we would work together to get me through this.

I got my injection of Neulastin the next day. That was one negative aspect of the bulk Taxotere treatment. However, there was nothing exciting to report about this visit. After a while, you go through the motions waiting, for it to be over. The process really makes you question your rigor.

I did have the diarrhea and vomiting for a few days after the treatment. At least I was prepared for it. Now, I just had to wait and see whether my body could rebound from the bulk treatment in a timely manner.

My white blood cell count was fine on June 11. I couldn't believe it. My red blood cell count was slightly low though.

A few days later, the skin around my port was very warm—hot, in fact—and very red. I made an appointment with the oncologist for June 18. At the appointment, my white blood cell count was fine, and I had lost two pounds within the past two weeks. They looked at the port and determined it was infected, but we didn't know how or why it got that way. They prescribed Augmentin, and it cleared up the infection quickly.

It appeared that my body was rebounding quicker, so I thought I could continue with the bulk treatments. I agreed to come back for the third, but I again told the oncologist that I wouldn't commit to anything afterward.

On June 21, a Monday, I was up one pound at my weigh-in, but I didn't let that get me down. My white blood cell count was on the high side at 9.5, but it was below the upper-limit of 10.2, so I could have the second bulk Taxotere treatment. The nurse couldn't find the freezy spray at first, and she asked if that was okay. I said that it definitely was not okay, so she searched and finally found it. They froze my port, and then I was on my way with my treatment. I went back the next day for my Neulastin injection, and again the same lovely side effects occurred.

Now I only had one more bulk treatment to go, and that actually seemed doable. I was finally seeing the end of chemotherapy, and I couldn't wait.

I had my six-month follow-up visit with the surgeon on June 25. All was well, and both Barbaras were happy to see me. They were so friendly, caring, and genuine. The one who had had breast cancer and I always hugged each other.

That week, my white blood cell count was slightly higher than the upper limit 10.9 versus 10.2. My red blood cell count, however, was slightly low at 3.74 compared to 4.04. I did not have to have any injections though.

On July 5, I noticed that my port was getting infected again. Really! I think that my body was trying to tell me that enough was enough.

When I went to the oncologist on July 6, my white blood cell count was still 0.6 too high. I had also gained three pounds, and this was the last weigh-in I tracked. During my whole treatment, I lost a total of seven pounds. Now you may ask, "Why on earth did you track your weight all that time for a change of just seven pounds?" I'll tell you why: It gave me something to focus on that was important to me. I wasn't going to let cancer stop me from achieving my existing goal of losing weight.

They prescribed more Augmentin, and I did not have a fever, so I was able to have the third bulk treatment of Taxotere. Unfortunately, they had to use my arm instead of my port due to the infection. After the appointment, I thought, *Yes, I'm finished! That was my last chemo treatment!*

I had my last Neulastin shot the next day. Yippee! The feeling of getting through all of the chemo sessions was indescribable. A huge weight was lifted off my shoulders. I had the normal unpleasant side effects, but I was glad to know that it would be my last instance of those too. Next stop, radiology!

Chapter 29

The Radiologist

On July 13, I stopped at the oncologist's office first, to have my blood work done, and then I went down the block to meet with the radiologist and discuss the next phase of my treatment. We discussed two options:

1. Radiate just the right breast (tumor area)
2. Radiate the right breast (tumor area) and the arm-pit (lymph node area)

The drawback of radiating my arm-pit was that it could cause a greater chance of lymphedema occurring. The radiologist said if four of my lymph nodes had been involved, he would have wanted to radiate my arm-pit. But with only three affected, it was a borderline case. In the end, I opted to only radiate the breast. This was something I had a choice in, so of course I chose the option that was different than the doctor's recommendation. I joke about being a rebel, but I did seriously stop and think about the choice I had to make.

While I was there, I got marked so that the radiologist would know exactly where to line up the machines at each treatment appointment. This helped minimize the residual radiation impact to my lungs. They line you up, mark you with a marker, and take a practice shot without the radiation to see that everything is set up properly. Then they tattoo the marks to make them permanent. I have one of these in the middle of my chest and one under my right arm. The process didn't really hurt.

They just felt like small pinches. I would have the marks forever as a permanent reminder of 2004. However, I knew that I had the power to choose the emotion that went along with this reminder. I could choose to remember it as the awful thing that happened to me in 2004 or as a time of triumph, in which I am a survivor. I chose the latter.

Chapter 30

The Final Surgery

The Augmentin prescription did not clear up the infection in my port this time. I took my second sick day on July 15 because I was scheduled to have the portacath removed. It's unusual to undergo surgery if you have a fever and infection, but because the device was causing the issues, they proceeded in this case. The aftereffects of removing the port were nowhere near as painful as when I had it installed. I again remembered to request the anti-nausea medicine.

This surgery was another item completed on my treatment checklist, and that put me another step closer to putting this portion of my life behind me. I continued to do everything I could to ensure that I didn't miss it.

As of July 16, all of my chemotherapy treatment was done, my port was removed, I had finished my antibiotics, and I had a new drain. The following Monday, July 19, I had my post-operative appointment with the surgeon. Everything looked good, and he removed the drain. That step also went much smoother than when I had the port implanted. I was really starting to enjoy these experiences that were more positive.

After this, I went to the oncologist's office once a week to get the CBC (blood work) done and take the results to the radiologist's office so that they could monitor my blood cell counts during my six weeks of daily treatments there. It actually took longer to get undressed and dressed at the radiologist than it did to get zapped.

Chapter 31

The Radiation—Summary Version

I have no notes about my radiation treatments other than the initial visit and the dates that I went for the weekly CBC tests at the oncology office (July 19 and 26 and August 2, 9, 17, 23, and 30). I was lucky in that my skin did not burn, dry out, or peel, all of which were potential side effects. I was able to wear my bra without any discomfort. Those six weeks were probably the best way that I could have thought of to end my treatment.

After my chemotherapy was completed, my holistic appointments changed to focus more on maintenance, to ensure that my body was staying tuned up. I saw the practitioner on August 10, and we worked on my respiratory and immune systems, low blood cell counts, and my thymus as well as my spleen and lymph system via laser acupuncture. We also adjusted my supplement dosages as necessary.

My last radiation treatment was on Friday, September 3, 2004—just in time for me to host a Woo-Hoo, I'm done! party.

Chapter 32

The Woo-Hoo, I'm Done! Party—Moving On

I planned a huge party for Labor Day weekend and invited all of my family and friends who supported me through my cancer treatment. I made homemade pasta sauce from my grandmother's recipe to use in the chicken parmigiana I put together, and my family and friends brought side dishes, desserts, and other items. It was a joyous celebration of life, and we had a wonderful time together.

That fall, I participated in the annual Long Island Making Strides against Breast Cancer Walk at Jones Beach State Park for the first time. Everyone at my Woo-Hoo, I'm Done! party made a donation to my fund. I raised a lot of money that year.

At this point, my hair was coming back in, so my head was stubbly. Because of this, my wig got progressively more uncomfortable. I decided that starting the next week, I was no longer going to wear my wig at work. I started wearing hats that were like baseball caps but nicer looking. According to the dress code, we were technically not allowed to, but no one said anything to me about it. I did get a few odd looks though, especially from those who never knew that I had been undergoing treatment for breast cancer.

On September 28, I had an appointment with my holistic practitioner. We worked on my thyroid, thymus, spleen, lymph, and alkalinity to support my immune system and ensure that my overall health continued to improve. A month later, at my next appointment with him, I told him that I was feeling a bit fatigued because I wasn't allowed to drink coffee anymore; I mentioned that I had craved it from October through February. Besides not being good for people in general, caffeine is worse for someone who gets a lot of cysts and has had breast cancer. I asked if there was anything he could do to help me. He decided to perform a muscle test and said that I had an issue with my pineal gland. This gland typically absorbs the sunlight, and mine was not doing that. He asked me if I had heard about people who experience depression or those who use ultraviolet plant lights in the wintertime. I told him that I had, and he explained that it was because they are not absorbing the sunlight and all of its nutrients.

Now, the type of muscle test he performed has nothing do with a work out at the gym. Anyone can perform it. Two people stand facing each other less than an arm's length apart. The person being tested sticks his or her dominant arm straight out to the side, parallel to the floor. The person doing the test puts a hand on the shoulder of the arm that isn't raised and the other hand on top of the hand on the outstretched arm. The person doing the test then pushes down on the other person's outstretched arm while he or she tries to keep it raised. At this point, the arm should stay parallel to the floor.

If the person being tested thinks that he or she has an allergy or an issue with a food or medicine, he or she would take that specific item in the non-dominant hand and hold it against his or her stomach. Then the person doing the testing would push down on the outstretched arm, as in the previous test. If the person cannot hold up the arm, his or her body does have an issue with that item and should avoid it.

When the holistic practitioner muscle tested my pineal gland, he put his fingers on my forehead between my eyes, by the bridge of my nose, and then he pushed on my arm. My arm went almost straight down to my side even though I tried really hard to hold it up. It was amazing.

He performed laser acupuncture and prescribed a pineal supplement. In just a few days, I felt great. I no longer felt like I needed coffee, and I wasn't tired. He reviewed the dosage of my other supplements and adjusted them as necessary.

I couldn't recall exactly when I stopped wearing caps and started spiking my hair with gel. In order for me to remember things like this, I have to relate them to major life events like birthdays or holidays. I looked at my photo albums and saw that I was still wearing my cap for Megan's sixth birthday at the beginning of November 2004.

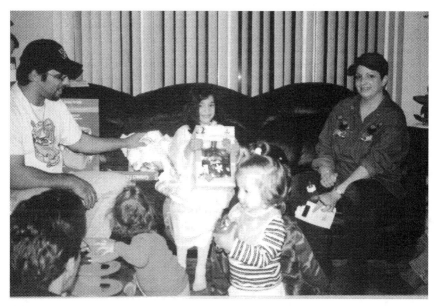

Megan's Sixth Birthday

Chapter 33

The Spa

My sister and I talked about getting away for a little spa weekend, and out of that conversation, another annual tradition was born. A group of us went to the Sagamore Inn located on the lake in Lake George, New York, for Veteran's Day weekend. I coordinated the entire event. It was absolutely beautiful there, and our spa services were amazing! I had the most relaxing massage that worked out the stress of the past ten months, and my facial made my skin glow. I really enjoyed my manicure and pedicure too. My hands and feet were in need of major pampering after all of the side effects of the chemotherapy. This was in fact the weekend that I started spiking the small amount of hair I had.

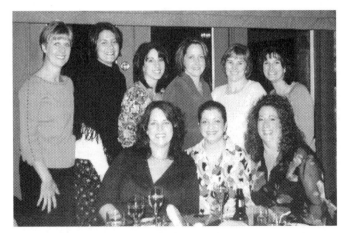

Spa Weekend

Chapter 34

The Year-End: I Made It!

On November 24, I had my annual mammogram and sonogram. They noted an eight-millimeter cyst in my left breast at the two o'clock position that they deemed suspicious. I thought, *Happy Thanksgiving to me! Here we go again. I just finished all my treatments a couple of months ago. Is this really happening?*

I followed up with the oncologist and the surgeon, and we all decided that no additional action was needed at the time. I should just keep my scheduled appointment with the surgeon in December. Even so, I was still apprehensive. It felt like the longest month ever waiting for the follow-up appointment.

On December 18, I met with my holistic practitioner, and he worked on my lymph system, thymus, spleen, and pineal gland as well as building up my blood counts. He adjusted the quantities of my supplements and kept me on the antivirals.

I went to the surgeon for my regular office visit. He reviewed the mammography and sonogram results from November and said that everything looked fine. He told me that our visits would now only be twice a year, and he'd see me again in six months. Yes! I was finally going to have fewer doctor appointments. I was seriously ecstatic, especially, since I had been worrying about this particular visit since the end of November.

The rest of the holidays were quite uneventful in comparison to the whole past year.

Happy New Year! The year 2004 was now over, and I could move on with my life! I couldn't wait to see where 2005 would take me.

2005

Chapter 35

Spring

I went to see my holistic practitioner a few months later on March 8, 2005, for a spring checkup. He said that, overall, I was doing well, and my body was rebounding nicely. I was having an issue with my ear and my throat, and he determined that I had an ear infection. He adjusted the dosage of my supplements (folic acid, spleen; fish oil, thymus; Monolaurin and Crotalus A, ear infection; and Crotalus C for my throat).

Now it was time to give myself something good. Since John and I had not gone with my sister and her friends on the cruise in 2004, we made plans to get away in April. We went to the Sandals resort in the Bahamas for a long weekend, and the girls stayed with my parents. Megan was six and Emma was two years old. For the most part, they were good for my mom and dad, but they cried a lot because they missed us. I remember my mom saying that John and I were not allowed to go away again for a while, at least until the girls got older. I felt awful, but at the same time, the weather was gorgeous at the resort. It was very nice and relaxing. It felt nice to do something for myself for a change, to get away and really unwind. We mostly hung out at the pool and the beach, although we did take an excursion over to the Atlantis Hotel. There were so many beautiful things to see there.

Chapter 36

Checkup Time

I went back to see the holistic practitioner on April 26. He decided we should take a look at my emotions because I was a little out-of-whack. I had some resentment and other emotions that needed adjusting. He treated me for this via laser acupuncture. He also advised me to maintain the current levels of my other supplements.

On May 25, I went to see the oncologist for a checkup, and I felt good. He said that he wanted to see me every three or four months. I did not agree. I asked how every six months sounded since I wasn't taking any post cancer medication. He didn't really agree, but he still gave me a hug. In fact, he always gave me a hug when I saw him. I really liked having him as my doctor. I thought, *I am glad that I didn't go and get a second opinion like my siblings wanted me to when this all started.* I left the examining room that day and I made my next appointment for October, five months later.

I went to see my surgeon on July 1 for my semi-annual checkup. He said that everything looked good, and he'd see me in six months. That's the kind of doctor's visit that I liked to have.

On August 15, the holistic practitioner treated me for pink-eye. I was still having some issues with viruses, so he recommended boosting my immune system some more. He gave me antiviral supplements and colloidal silver drops. The latter burned but cleared up my eyes quickly. From that point on, I kept the drops on hand just in case my eyes ever started to feel weird.

Chapter 37

Family Focus

Although I haven't mentioned it a lot thus far, doing things with and for my daughters was another very important part of my life—a major distraction from "IT". I was one of Megan's Girl Scout Brownie leaders. We had a lot of fun with the other moms and girls in the troop. Emma was still very young at the time, so she was not involved in all of the extracurricular activities yet. I could probably sit down and write a book about each of my daughters and how important they are to me, but I'll just give you some of the highlights.

Megan was progressing well with her physical therapy, and someone recommended that we try hippo-therapy. That is where handicapped children ride horses and work on different things depending upon the disability. In Megan's case, we needed to work on her core for stability purposes. We took her for an evaluation at a facility that specialized in hippo-therapy. Her disability was not severe enough to qualify her for official hippo-therapy, but she could still participate in therapy on horses weekly. She really loved it. Megan also learned how to care for the horses.

When she started in September, Megan had three people guiding her: one on each side and another to lead the horse. By the summer of 2005, Megan was able to participate in competitions with one person on the side and one leading the horse. She got a blue ribbon at her first show! She participated in a few more shows and received blue and red ribbons. Eventually, she grew out of riding horses and embarked on other endeavors. I think that she realized that the horses were big, and accidents could happen when her pediatric orthopedist was accidently thrown from her horse and broke her back. The doctor healed, but I think that it had a definite impact on Megan's decision to stop riding.

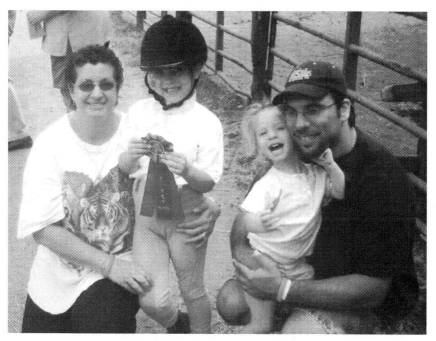

Megan's First Horse Show

Chapter 38

Fall Follow-Ups

I had my checkup with the oncologist on October 7, and he gave me a hug hello. Everything looked good, and I felt good. We talked about how I had been the past several months and what my girls were up to. It was nice to know that he cared, and he didn't' seem like he was in a rush to move on to the next patient. He gave me a prescription for my annual mammogram and sonogram. We discussed the timing of my next appointment. He wanted to see me in three to four months. I made my next appointment for March, five months later.

I went to see the holistic practitioner on October 17, and he worked on my lungs because I felt short of breath when I climbed the stairs at work. This was most likely a result of the radiation treatments, which did hit a small part of my lung. The oncologist had told me that these trailing symptoms might disappear over time.

On November 15, I had my mammogram and sonogram done. They noted a five-millimeter cyst in my left breast, located four-centimeters from the nipple at the 9 o'clock position, but it was deemed non-cancerous.

Yes, I had made it through another year! Happy New Year! Since 2005 went so well, I was looking forward to what 2006 would bring!

2006

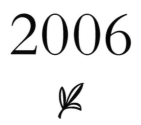

Chapter 39

The Psychic

I started off 2006 with a bang. On January 23, John, Megan, and I went to see Billy Joel in concert at Madison Square Garden. Before the concert, we went to Greenwich Village so that I could see a psychic who was recommended by someone at work. I don't know if you believe in such things, but he was able to tell me about so many things that were right on the mark about my family members, my life, and so on.

I did not tell him anything about my health or my family's health, but at one point during our session, he told me that I would be "prone to lumps and bumps that will prove to be nothing." I was very taken aback by this. I fessed up that I had breast cancer in 2004, so I didn't understand how what he said could be true. He then said that I wasn't listening to him. He repeated what he had said previously and clarified that his statement was for the future. In other words, he did not forecast any breast cancer in my future.

The psychic's statement, coupled with my holistic practitioner ridding my body of the adenovirus that we felt caused the cancer in the first place, aligned with my determination that this was a one-time occurrence in my life. I was free to have the most amazing time with my family as I watched my favorite musician at my daughter's first concert!

I had a feeling that this would be the best year in a while for me.

Chapter 40

New Year, New Appointments

I went to my semi-annual checkup with the surgeon on January 26. As usual, I was greeted by the two Barbaras. We spoke about the holidays and how we were all feeling. The doctor was happy that everything looked good, and he sent me away, saying that he'd see me again in six months.

On February 14, I went to see the holistic practitioner for a recheck of my thymus, spleen, blood, auto immune system, and pH levels, as well as the amounts of vitamins, fish oil, and folic acid I was taking. Overall, I was doing great, and we just needed to adjust my dosages.

I had my semi-annual checkup with my oncologist on March 13. Everything looked good, and I told him that I had been feeling well. We caught up, and I got my semi-annual hug. I reminded him that I was not taking any medication other than my holistic supplements, and he didn't push the three-to-four month time-frame for the next appointment.

I saw the holistic practitioner again for a quick check on April 14. Everything looked good with my thymus, spleen, blood, and immune systems. And I felt great!

I was seeing some type of doctor every month, and from my notes everything was going great and I was happy. I would attribute this feeling to my wellness and the good news. So far, 2006 was going along very smoothly. I decided that I would start grouping my appointments together so that I could get back to a more normal lifestyle.

Soon it was time to make a different kind of appointment. I needed to do something with my hair. When it grew back in, it came back with Shirley Temple curls from the chemotherapy. This was called chemo-curl. I would pull on the curls to straighten them out, and they would bounce right back. I went to see Sal, and we came up with a plan. He did a chemical treatment that pulled all of the curl out of my hair to make it more manageable. It looked great for a month or two, and then it curled right back up. Sal gave my hair another chemical treatment and left it on longer. This time, it worked! My hair went back to the way it was before I had cancer.

Chapter 41

Casting for Recovery

I experienced the most wonderful and therapeutic retreat in June 2006. My sister-in-law had told me about a weekend organized and run by a non-profit organization called Casting for Recovery (http:// castingforrecovery.org/). It costs no money for survivors of breast cancer, and it is meant to provide women with powerful tools to overcome the challenges they face. The organization was having a retreat locally, and space was limited, so I filled out an application promptly, and it was accepted.

On May 15, I asked my oncologist if he would complete a medical release form for my participation in the retreat.

The weekend of the retreat, I met other women who were survivors just like me, and we all shared our different experiences and stories. At one of the ceremonies, we each had to choose a rock for positive energy. I still carry my rock in my wallet.

I also learned how to fly fish that weekend. First we learned on land, and then we went and fished in a river at a state park. The organizers made sure that we each got the experience of catching and releasing at least one fish. It is the most peaceful experience. You put waders on and stand in the river. Everything is so quiet. You hear water rushing and birds chirping. You take the fishing rod and flick it back and forth. Success in fly-fishing is all in your wrist. Each of us got to take home our own fly-fishing rod and reel that had been donated by a local company. I would recommend that you look into

Casting for Recovery, and if you qualify, participate in one of these retreats. If you do not qualify, they are always looking for volunteers and donations to help support their cause and give back to other breast cancer survivors.

Chapter 42

The Scare, Part I

My next six-month checkups with the surgeon and the oncologist were both on August 4, and both visits went well. There were no issues during the prior six months. I felt good as well. I was in and out of both appointments fairly quickly. I got to catch up with the two Barbaras at the surgeon's office, and I got a hug from my oncologist. I also got the prescription for my annual mammogram and sonogram. I waited for a December appointment because I wanted to have both tests done during one visit, and that was the first time that they could schedule it.

On August 22, I had my periodic check with my holistic practitioner, and all of my dosages remained the same.

I had my annual mammogram and sonogram done on December 27. I have a note that I got a call from the oncologist right away. There was a new cyst located at three o'clock, five centimeters from the nipple in the right breast. It measured five by four by four millimeters, and he suggested that I follow up with the surgeon. I remember this one clearly because I did not tell a soul about this phone call. I kept it to myself, as I didn't want to worry anyone.

Due to the holidays, I couldn't get an appointment with the surgeon until early January. I was very disappointed about this delay and it felt like déjà vu.

This was not a happy New Year for me, but I tried to maintain my optimism about what 2007 would have in store for me.

2007

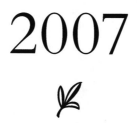

Chapter 43

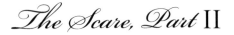

On January 8, 2007, I went to see the surgeon, and he performed a fine-needle aspiration and sent it off to be analyzed. When I first met him back in 2004 and he saw my original tumor, he was very sure about my diagnosis before he even performed the biopsy. This time, he didn't seem overly concerned, so I wasn't either. I left the office not thinking much more about it.

On January 15, I received a phone call saying that the results came back inconclusive. I needed to go back for an actual biopsy. I couldn't get another appointment until January 26. I again did not tell anyone at home or at work. I felt like I was going to lose my mind. I asked Barbara to change my contact information to my cell phone number. I didn't want the surgeon's office to leave a message at my home because I didn't want my family to know what was going on. I didn't want to tell anyone anything, because I didn't know anything conclusive, and I didn't want to worry them if it turned out to be nothing. So, it was my secret burden starting at the end of December. This was one of the most difficult times in my life. I couldn't believe it was happening. It felt like the bad dream from three years ago was repeating itself almost to the day. What a nightmare!

I was very agitated, worried, and upset when I went to my appointment with the surgeon on January 26. He performed a fine-needle biopsy and sent it out for analysis. He again didn't seem overly concerned, but I felt much less confident this time. I had to wait another week before I heard anything.

I saw the oncologist for my regular five-month month checkup on January 27. Other than the pending results from the biopsy, nothing was new. But I think that was enough for the beginning of the year.

On February 2, I got a call from the surgeon as I pulled into my driveway after work. He let me know that the results were in and everything was fine. I was happy and relieved, and I told him that if we ever had to do this again, he needed to do both tests at once because there was no way that I could go through this whole waiting game again.

I saw the surgeon on April 13 as a follow up to the biopsies. Everything looked good, and we moved back to semi-annual checkups.

Chapter 44

More Health Issues, More Surgery

At the same time as the scare with the lump and biopsy, I was also experiencing some female issues. I made an appointment with my ob-gyn, and after some tests, they determined that I had a fairly large cyst on one of my ovaries that was causing me a lot of problems. We discussed my options and decided that the best course of action, given my medical history and the fact that I did not plan to have more children, was for me to have a hysterectomy. There was a lot of debate on whether to have a full hysterectomy or to leave the other ovary intact. I preferred for them to take everything, but they wanted to leave the one ovary. We made a deal before the surgery. When they got in there, if the other ovary looked bad, they would remove it, but if it looked okay, they would biopsy it so that I would have peace of mind. It was a laparoscopic surgery, and I had a really good recovery. They left the one ovary, and the biopsy results came back normal.

On May 30, I went to my holistic practitioner because I was having a difficult time with my allergies. The over-the-counter medicine was not working, and I was miserable. He treated me for fifty-eight different pollens and grasses. He also worked on boosting my spleen, maintaining my immune system, increasing my blood cell counts, and maintaining my alkalinity. I told him about my hysterectomy so that he could ensure that all of my hormones were in balance. After he treated me with laser acupuncture for the allergies, I was not allowed to be outside for the next twenty-five hours so that the treatment would be effective. Within forty-eight hours, I no longer needed over-the-counter allergy medicine.

Chapter 45

Helpless

During the summer of 2007 my daughter Megan, who was eight years old, came to me and told me that she wanted to be normal. At the time, Megan was upset that she couldn't run around my parents' yard like her cousins. She told me that she wanted to be on one of those TV shows where people got makeovers or new houses, and their situation was better by the end of the episode. Megan even asked me if God or Santa Claus could make her normal. All I could do was cry and hold her as I felt helpless.

I mentioned an option she had that was called heel cord surgery. She said she wanted to have it, and I tried to explain to her that there was no guarantee that the surgery would make her normal. Her response, at eight years old, was, "I am willing to take that risk."

Megan has always been very mature and smart, but I was shocked to hear that come out of her mouth. I told her that I would call her pediatric orthopedist to discuss the possibilities of the operation further. The next day, I told the doctor about Megan's wishes, and together we decided that Megan would have the operation in December, right before Christmas break, so that she would have more time to heal at home. I told Megan about this plan. She was very excited but also disappointed that she had to wait a few months.

Chapter 46

Semi-Annual Check

On August 27, I had a follow-up appointment with my holistic practitioner. It was a straightforward visit. My allergy issues had cleared up right after the May visit, and all of my other systems and test results were unchanged. Finally, my body had some homeostasis!

After this appointment, I reduced the frequency of the holistic visits, but I continued taking the supplements. I knew that was important. When I needed to see him for a specific issue later, he had gotten so busy that I could not get an appointment with him. I decided to change to the practitioner who had treated and trained the man I was originally seeing. My main issues for the next few years were related to allergies and occasional viruses, so I would go to get treated for these as needed.

I saw both my surgeon and my oncologist on November 2 for my semi-annual checkups. I got my customary hug from the oncologist and from Barbara at the surgeon's office. It was a great feeling to hug another survivor and congratulate each other on another six months of wellness. Both appointments went well that day, and I was in and out of their offices fairly quickly.

Chapter 47

Megan's Surgery

On December 11, John and I took Megan to her heel cord surgery. She looked so cute in the hospital gown and cap. She was very nervous as she sat in a reclining chair in the private pre-surgical waiting room. They gave her some medicine to relax her, and when it kicked in Megan got very silly and slurred her words like she was drunk. John and I laughed our butts off—sorry, Megan.

Megan's pediatric orthopedist performed the surgery. She opened the back of Megan's right leg just above her heel and made several angled cuts in the heel cord. After the surgery, her leg was put in a cast to keep her foot at a ninety-degree angle while it healed. The hope was that when Megan healed, she would be able to keep her heel flat on the ground at all times rather than standing on her toes.

The surgery went well, and the doctor was very optimistic about the long-term effects.

Chapter 48

Happy New Year!

I had my annual mammogram and sonogram on December 15. The results for both were clear, with no abnormalities noted. Thank goodness!

Merry Christmas and happy New Year to me! I actually made it through 2007. I was very glad that the year ended on a better note than it started on, and I was looking forward to 2008!

2008

Chapter 49

Sharing and Support

Teresa, a friend in my department at work, stopped by my desk in March to talk to me. I knew she had something specific on her mind. She was not the first person to stop by and ask, "Would you mind if we talked?" Other women had done the same, talking with me about their questions and concerns when they too were diagnosed with breast cancer.

Teresa and I had worked together while I was going through my breast cancer treatment, and she had just been diagnosed with thyroid cancer. She had two small daughters and was feeling overwhelmed. We discussed her concerns and her options. She asked me about what I had gone through and how I managed. From that point on, we were confidants for each other.

I know how hard it was for people to talk to me because I could not get myself to talk to anyone else. Maybe it was easier for them than talking to a complete stranger. The only person that I knew with breast cancer was my friend who was only in the beginning stages of her treatment when I was diagnosed, and her doctor's approach was totally different than mine.

On May 9, I had my semi-annual checkups with the surgeon and oncologist. Both visits went well. I was given the seal of approval and went on my way for another six months.

Chapter 50

Bullying and Promoting Disability Awareness

Late spring 2008 brought about some new challenges with Megan and how we dealt with her cerebral palsy. She was in the fourth grade at this time, and she started to complain about pain in her right leg. If we touched it, she cried hysterically. I was at a loss as to what to do, so I took her to the emergency room twice within ten days for them to look at her leg. She said that she needed a cast or crutches, but the doctors could find nothing wrong.

Megan finally discussed things calmly with me, and I found out that field day was coming up at school. She felt that she could not participate—no one wanted her on their team. The kids were saying things about her that upset her. I was very upset that her peers were bullying her. She started seeing the school counselor to see if they could get things resolved in school.

I started doing research, and within two weeks, I had a binder full of information on programs that the school could use to educate the children and the staff about various disabilities. Most of the programs were either free or of minimal expense. I presented the binder to the pupil personnel services department, which managed the care of children with special needs in the whole school district. I didn't get very far, so I decided to work directly with Megan's school to help her directly. The school worked with me and started bringing in groups to educate the children about disability awareness and treating all people equally and with respect.

My mother and I started a non-profit corporation called Sensitivity Awareness Inc., but my full-time job and other volunteer obligations kept us from spending a lot of time getting the organization up and running. We have kept the corporation alive by submitting all of the necessary annual filings, but it's not currently active. Maybe in the future we will get the organization running and be able to help other children. In the meantime, I always make sure that Megan is protected and getting everything that she needs.

Chapter 51

Positive Direction

Megan had joined the school chorus at the beginning of fourth grade. She really enjoyed it. She almost got a solo for the spring concert, but it went to a fifth grader who was graduating. Megan's chorus teacher told me that she thought that Megan was a really good singer, and I asked if she had any recommendations for a voice teacher. She recommended a music teacher from one of the other elementary schools who lived near my home and gave private lessons.

The following July, Megan started weekly piano lessons from this teacher with a small concentration on voice lessons. Megan picked up the piano very quickly, and we bought a piano so that she could practice at home. The music teacher told me that Megan had an amazing ear, but she shouldn't rely on that alone. Musicians need to be able to read music, or they can only progress to a certain point. We made sure that Megan practiced piano all of the time.

September 2008 was a fun time! Emma started kindergarten, and Megan entered fifth grade. I was going to be a Girl Scout leader for both Emma's Daisy Troop and Megan's Girl Scout Junior Troop. I was amazed that I could fit all of this in and still work full-time. It was like the saying, "If you want something done, give it to a busy person."

Chapter 52

Four-Year Follow-Up

On November 21, I went to the surgeon for my semi-annual checkup and told him about a cyst that was causing me some pain in my left breast. He used a sonogram machine and performed a fine-needle aspiration and biopsy. He thought that everything was fine, but he sent them out for analysis. I was a little nervous in light of my past history, but I tried not to dwell on it.

My surgeon moved me to annual checkups. It was a surprise to me, but now I only needed to see him once a year. I got my hug from Barbara and wished her well for the coming year.

I had my semi-annual checkup with my oncologist on November 21. I told him about my appointment with the surgeon but he did not want to change to annual appointments. He gave me a prescription for my annual mammogram and sonogram, and I got my hug and was on my way.

On November 28, the surgeon called to let me know that the biopsy results were back, and everything was fine. Phew! I could breathe a little easier after that news.

Chapter 53

The Call—Again

On December 24, I had my annual mammogram and sonogram. A few days later, I got a call from the oncology office.

The reports were good, but there were two small cysts in my left breast. Both were located at about four o'clock, and both were about 0.7 centimeters. No further tests were needed at this time, but I should have a follow-up sonogram in approximately six months. The oncologist said that his office would mail me a prescription for it, and I should make an appointment for next year.

So, 2008 had come to an end. Happy New Year! I was glad to make it through another year and see what 2009 brought.

2009

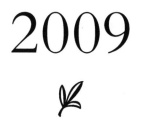

Chapter 54

Life Takes Over

A lot of wonderful things happened in my family at the beginning of 2009. I've always tried to focus on their needs and give them all of the opportunities possible to excel

Megan's piano and voice lessons were progressing very well. She was getting ready to participate in her first New York State School Music Association (NYSSMA) solo competition. At this event, a person performs his or her musical talent—in this case, singing, in front of a judge alone or with an accompanist if needed. The performer is judged on things like pronunciation, tone, tempo, and the like. She sang a level two piece and scored twenty-six out of twenty-eight which translated to a score of outstanding. I was so proud of her!

Megan was also nominated and subsequently chosen to participate in SCMEA, the Suffolk County Music Educators Association. Based on nominations from music teachers and students' NYSSMA scores, the association selects just a few people from each school to participate in an all-county performance. We were all so excited for her to participate in such a prestigious program. The students learned the songs on their own time and only got together three times to practice as a group. The concert was absolutely amazing! They sounded like a professional group that had been singing together for a long time.

On May 28, I had my follow-up sonogram, and the cysts that were noted on the report from the December 24 exam were either unchanged or decreased in size. This was a good report!

The year flew by. That spring, Megan was finishing up fifth grade and getting ready to graduate, so I was dealing with the school district to ensure that she'd be safe in the middle school. Emma was finishing her first year of kindergarten and having a great year making new friends. She enjoyed learning things in school and with her Girl Scout troop.

In the latter half of 2009, Megan was adjusting to middle school. I was meeting with teachers regularly and still running both Girl Scout troops.

If you have been keeping track, you will realize that I didn't mention going to any regular checkups during 2009. I actually didn't make any appointments during this year. I don't know what happened. I think that I may have thought that the follow-up in May was as a result of my regular checkup with my doctors, but it was not. Oops!

The whole year went by and I did not have one single doctor appointment aside from the sonogram in May. I got caught up in my life!

Happy New Year to me! I made it through 2009 with hardly any doctor appointments. I'm not recommending that you follow in my footsteps, but sometimes life just happens. Now on to 2010!

2010

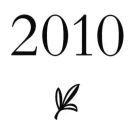

Chapter 55

Focus on the Children

January 2010 rolled around, and I made all of my appointments for one day in February. My last visit to the oncologist and surgeon had been in May 2009.

Megan was nominated and accepted for SCMEA again—we were so excited. They only picked three sixth graders for the choral group, and Megan was one of them. What a boost to her self-esteem this was!

Chapter 56

Its About Time

On the morning of February 12, I went to see my surgeon. Barbara was still doing well, and we gave each other our usual hug. All looked good, but the surgeon still wanted to see me in six months. *Well I guess that is the penalty I get for skipping a year*, I thought. I immediately made my follow-up appointment for August.

My oncologist appointment went well, other than him scolding me for missing a whole year. He wanted to see me in six months as well, but their calendar only went out to April, so I had to make a note to follow up and make an appointment for August. I got my hug and prescriptions for my blood work and annual mammography and sonogram.

I went and got my blood work done right away since I had some time. I had to get my blood work done at a separate lab now in order for it to be covered by health insurance.

That afternoon, I went to the ob-gyn and had my annual checkup. I had missed this appointment as well the year before.

Next, I went to the holistic practitioner, and it went well. He said I had an overall rating of two, which is a great score, very healthy (only a one would be better, but that's a very hard score to get). We adjusted my supplements slightly.

By the end of the day, I was exhausted. I know that I am great with time management, but five appointments in one day was a little much.

I had my mammogram and sonogram on February 15 and waited for the call that I just knew was going to come a few days later.

Chapter 57

The Calls

Late in the afternoon on February 17, I got the usual call from the oncology office. The oncologist said that the report for the mammography came back fine. The sonogram report stated that I was very cystic overall and that there was a mass measuring 0.4 centimeters in my left breast at the five o'clock position. This mass was new compared to prior sonograms. It was deemed suspicious, and the radiologist recommended that it should be biopsied. *Here we go again!* The oncologist was going to send me a copy of the written report from the radiologist, and he also recommended a follow-up sonogram in six months.

On February 18, I called the surgeon's office first thing in the morning and asked for an appointment for Friday, February 19 (since he only had office hours on Mondays and Fridays). However, he was on a cruise, so I couldn't get an appointment until the next Monday afternoon to have the biopsy performed.

A little later on February 18, the ob-gyn office called to let me know that my Pap test came back with some abnormal cells. The test for HPV was negative, so the abnormal cells might just be as a result of my body fighting an infection. They asked me to come back in three months to repeat the test.

I was freaking out a little bit, so I sent an instant message to Teresa, my friend at work. I told her what was going on and that I was worried. She was there for me, and I felt a lot better after confiding in her. Even though "IT" had been out of my life now for a few years, the waiting did not get any easier. And the calls from the doctors didn't help. Sometimes it is much easier to talk to someone who's been there. Teresa assured me that everything was going to be okay. I waited and worried all weekend while I took care of my family.

On February 22, I went to have the biopsy done. The surgeon sent out the samples for testing, and I was on pins and needles for the next week waiting for the results. Barbara gave me a supportive hug. When the results came back about a week later, everything was fine—no cancer. He wanted to see me back again in six weeks.

As soon as I got the good news about the test results, I told Teresa. We were both very excited and relieved.

I had a follow-up appointment with the surgeon on April 2. Everything still looked good, thank goodness! Barbara and I gave each other a celebratory hug. After so many visits to the same doctors, they almost become a part of your family. This is especially true when the staff has remained the same over the years.

Chapter 58

Megan's Singing

In May, Megan participated in the NYSSMA solo competition again. She performed a level three solo and scored a twenty-five out of twenty-eight which translated to a score of excellent. She was disappointed that she didn't do as well as the prior year. However, I told her that it took a lot of courage to sing in front of a judge, and she should be proud of how she did. It was another great performance for my little singer!

Her private teacher said that Megan was progressing so well with her vocals that it was time to move on to a new teacher who was a voice major. Her current teacher was a piano major with a voice minor. The new vocal coach was a friend of the piano teacher, so we made the switch and started to work solely on Megan's singing.

Chapter 59

More Follow-Ups

On July 7, I had my follow-up sonogram per the radiologist's recommendation at my February 15 sonogram. The results stated that the nodule at five o'clock remained unchanged and demonstrated benign features. They recommended another follow-up in six months.

At my six-month follow-up appointment with my surgeon on August 13, he finally said that I didn't have to see him anymore as long as I kept seeing the oncologist and ob-gyn. I was ecstatic! But I mentioned that based on my history, I'd most likely end up seeing him at least once a year after my mammogram and sonogram because there was usually something they needed to take a closer look at.

On November 2, I went to see my oncologist. He wasn't happy that I hadn't seen him since February, and I explained to him that I had an appointment scheduled in September but had to cancel it because I was sick. I couldn't get another appointment that fit my schedule until November. He didn't really like that reason, but other than that, the visit went well. I let him know that the surgeon had signed off on me, and I didn't need to see him anymore as long as I kept my other regular appointments. I was supposedly still on a semi-annual schedule with the oncologist, but I convinced him to move our visits to an annual basis. I got my hug and I was on my way.

This was great news to end 2010! Happy New Year! After six years I finally felt like I was moving forward, medically speaking. I was looking forward to 2011.

2011

Chapter 60

Disappointment of a Child

In January 2011, Megan was in seventh grade and again nominated for SCMEA, but she was not selected this year. Megan was very, very upset, so I tried to reassure her. I explained that they only picked a few children from each school and that she should feel lucky for being picked two years in a row. It didn't appear to help her much, but I tried to be as supportive as I could.

Singing was the closest activity Megan had to a sport, so this loss could be equated to an athlete losing a big playoff game.

Chapter 61

Biopsy

On March 17, I went back to my original holistic practitioner, as the team I had seen for the past few years had recently relocated out of the area. He and I spoke about the stress I was under at work, and he worked on my neurotransmitters and emotions. I needed a calcium-magnesium supplement, and my trace minerals were low. He also gave me a colostrum supplement to help support my immune system.

On April 5, I had my annual mammogram and sonogram. I got the results in the mail a week or so later. The sonogram results stated that the nodule in my left breast from July 7, 2010, had increased slightly and showed a slight irregularity in its margins. A core needle biopsy was recommended. The mammography results stated that additional views of a 1.1 centimeter round nodule in my right breast were needed.

I was a little upset about this. I had thought that since I didn't get a call, everything was okay and the letters were just a formality. I called the radiology office as soon as I got the letters and expressed my rage and frustration. They apologized and said that they did not know why I never got a phone call. The radiologist was able to get me in for the additional views of the right breast on April 14. I again didn't get a call, but I could not get comfortable until I received the letter. The results stated that the nodule was benign.

On April 29, the surgeon reviewed the films from my most recent mammogram and the two sets of sonograms and decided that there was no need for a biopsy at this time. I joked with him about what I had said the August before, and now there I was. We agreed that I should have follow-up scans done in six months as a precaution.

Chapter 62

Positive Feedback

In May, Megan performed a level four piece for the NYSSMA solo competition and scored a twenty-seven out of twenty-eight which translated to a score of outstanding. The songs were getting more difficult, her self-confidence was improving, and her scores were staying consistent! She's amazing, and I am so proud of her.

Megan's voice coach told us about another singing group that Megan could get involved with. It was called the Metropolitan Youth Orchestra (MYO). They had started in Nassau County and were slowly growing. They had different levels of orchestra and choral groups, depending upon the children's skill and grade level.

Megan had to audition in front of two conductors from MYO. A few weeks later, we got a letter inviting her to join their ensemble. She graciously accepted. This group met one evening a week during the school year and performed concerts at various venues: the Stahler Center at Stony Brook University, Adelphi University, Hofstra University, Queens College, and Carnegie Hall, just to name a few. The sound quality of the singers was very similar to that of the SCMEA groups. These children sang and played their instruments not because they were forced to, but because it was their passion, and the resulting sounds were astounding.

Chapter 63

Health Check

On October 10, I had my six-month follow-up mammogram and sonogram. The mammography came back clear, and the sonogram showed an area that the radiologist believed to be benign. Radiology recommended that I have another follow-up in six months to confirm that the area had not changed.

Happy New Year—2011 has ended! My overall health was good, but I realized that I forgot to make an appointment with the oncologist this year. One daughter would be starting high school in the fall, and the other would be going into fourth grade! I thought 2012 was going to be a very interesting year.

2012

Chapter 64

More Disappointments for Megan

In January, Megan was in the middle of eighth grade, and she was again nominated for SCMEA. Sadly, she again was not selected to participate. She was a little less disappointed this time around. Maybe this was because she was growing up and realizing that it was an honor to be nominated, or maybe it was because she had gotten involved with the Metropolitan Youth Orchestra.

Chapter 65

No Changes

On April 3, I went to the oncologist for my follow-up appointment. I got yelled at because I had not seen him since November 2010. Other than that, things went well, and he agreed that we could stay on the annual schedule as long as I actually made and kept the appointments. He gave me a light smack on the shoulder and then my usual hug.

I had my annual mammogram and sonogram on April 7. The results for both were normal with no suspicious findings.

That same month, on April 13, I saw my surgeon. I know we supposedly stopped the annual visits, but since I was there the year before as a result of my new mammogram and sonogram we somehow restarted the annual follow-ups. I didn't mind going to the surgeon's office. I got to see how Barbara was doing, and we got to catch up on things. The visit went well, and we parted ways, hopefully for another year.

Chapter 66

More Positivity

In May, Megan again participated in the NYSSMA solo competition. She performed a level five piece and scored a ninety-eight out of one hundred which translated to a score of an "A+". As students progress to higher levels, the scoring is done at a much more granular level, and the judges look for progressive improvement in very particular skills. The songs and the skills involved to perform them are much more difficult. Megan continues to amaze me every year!

That June, Megan graduated from middle school fairly unscathed, and it was time to get ready for high school!

Over the summer Megan, her friend Nikki, Emma, and I went to Knoebels Amusement Resort with my friend Sharon and her family. Knoebels is a really cool amusement park in Pennsylvania with rides and attractions for all ages. The older girls went around by themselves, and Emma and I spent time with Sharon and her family. We definitely had a good time and wanted to make plans to go back the following year.

Chapter 67

High School and the Holidays

In September, Megan started high school. I made sure that I met with all of her teachers right away so that they were aware of her disability and her IEP (Individualized Education Plan) that provided her with certain accommodations (a special locker location, an elevator key, passing time in the hallway, etcetera).

The holidays were coming around again soon, and for the past two years, my daughter Emma had been asking Santa Claus for an archery set. This Christmas, my mom and dad gave her gift certificates so that she could try her hand at archery in the coming year. We had been trying to find an activity that Emma would enjoy getting involved with, but we hadn't had any luck as of yet. We were hoping that she would end up liking archery.

Happy New Year! Goodbye 2012 and hello 2013! It was an uneventful year in the health department, which was a good thing. It allowed me to focus on my daughters, whom I love more than anything. They have been very instrumental in keeping me focused on the future. I am thankful for both of them every day.

2013

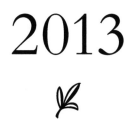

Chapter 68

The Bullying Continues

Ninth grade was very hard for Megan. She racked up a lot of absences during the first few months of school that fall for what I thought were valid reasons at the time. I didn't realize what was actually going on until January 2013.

She was getting bullied at school about her disability, and it was a very tough time for us. As soon as I was aware of what was going on and the gravity of the situation, I immediately contacted the school district to work with them. I got Megan the help that she needed, and we moved forward. I want to treat this private matter with discretion and sensitivity, but I learned that sometimes we parents don't really see what's going on with our children. I've been paying much more attention since this situation.

Megan's cerebral palsy is always going to be her cross to bear. We all have things we will have to face in our lives. By standing up and facing our challenges, we become stronger, more compassionate people.

I am very proud of the fact that Megan was willing to do the work and get the help that she needed. Now she will be strong enough to handle herself when faced with any bullies in the future. There are always going to be people that don't understand why she walks differently and are too small-minded to see her for the wonderful young lady that she is. But I am confident that she will rise above and become even stronger. I was so proud of Megan that I surprised her with tickets to see her favorite performer, Justin Bieber. When I wrapped the tickets,

I made it a multi-step process for her to get to them. I took a video recording of her opening the tickets and going absolutely nuts. She was ecstatic. Before she saw them, she thought that I had gotten her One Direction tickets because I was giving her a lot of directions in order to get to the gift.

I mentioned to a friend at work the challenges Megan was facing and how I had given her the concert tickets. My friend was astonished and appalled that the other students would act that way in this day and age. And then she thought that my packaging was funny. She told me that she knew someone that might be able to actually get me two tickets to see One Direction. I was so surprised, and I knew that there were no guarantees because the concert sold out a year in advance. Well, she was able to get the tickets, so Emma helped me set up another surprise for Megan. I did a little deceitful packaging, and we recorded the whole thing again. I thought Megan was going to pass out with utter joy and excitement. I took the video to work and showed it to my friend who got me the tickets. Megan thanked her over and over in the video.

Chapter 69

The Accomplishments

On an even more positive note, Megan was nominated for SCMEA and selected this time. It was some good news during a really tough time, but the excitement soon wore off because Megan got a really bad cold. Since they only rehearsed as a group three times, they were not allowed to miss any rehearsals. Because of Megan's illness, she was not able to participate in the actual concert. I still ordered the CD though because the music was always so beautiful.

In March, Megan made her Carnegie Hall debut with the Metropolitan Youth Orchestra. It was one of the most amazing concerts at one of the most amazing venues in the world. I even got her accomplishment posted on our school district's electronic bulletin board. This made some of her peers take notice of her singing talent. Kids at school went up to her and said that they hadn't realized that she could sing. Even one of the cashiers in the lunch room recognized her name when Megan swiped her card to pay for lunch. This was the kind of positive attention my daughter needed.

Hauppauge's Electronic Bulletin Board

In February, Emma started her group archery lessons. She really liked it and was actually pretty good at it. She shot ten yards with a recurve bow and actually hit some bull's-eyes. She decided that this was something that she wanted to continue. We had finally found something that Emma could really get into!

I spoke to my family about Emma's growing love for archery, and they all agreed to chip in for a gift certificate so that Emma could get her own bow, arrows, and accessories for her birthday. When my mom bought the gift card, the clerk told her about a junior archery league that would start the week after Emma's birthday, so I signed her up as part of her birthday gift. Emma was very surprised.

We went to the archery store right away to make sure that Emma had all of her own equipment before the league started. She started shooting on April 19 with a score of ninety-one. Scoring works like this: There are ten ends (rounds), and an archer uses three arrows for each end. The bull's-eye is worth ten points, so the highest score possible per end is thirty. After all ten ends, the total possible perfect score is three hundred. She started taking individual lessons each week, and her skills and scores improved. By the end of the nine-week league she had shot a 207. She kept going to lessons through most of that summer.

Emma's Great Arrows

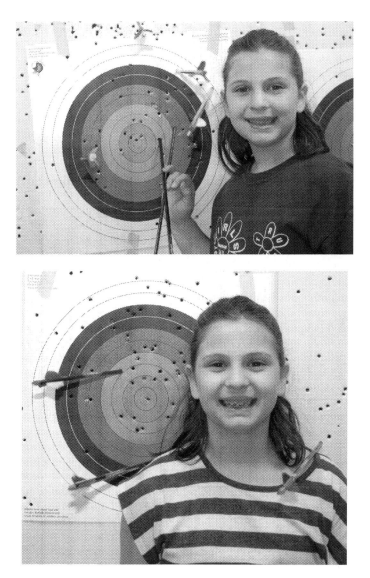

Chapter 70

No Call

On April 29, I had a full day of annual follow-up appointments, but this time I only scheduled three appointments in one day. I did the blood work and the ob-gyn visit on different days.

I went to see my surgeon and then my oncologist. Both of those visits went well, and we spoke about how the past year had gone. Both doctors gave me the thumbs-up for another year, and I got all of my usual hugs.

Later that afternoon, I had my annual mammogram and sonogram. I did not get one of those phone calls with bad news. I got my results like anyone else would, in a letter dated May 1, 2013, stating that my results were normal, and that there was no evidence of any suspicious findings! Yippee! That made me very happy. After nine years, it was such a great feeling to complete all of my appointments and tests without any surprises.

Chapter 71

More Great Family News

Megan performed a level six piece at the NYSSMA solo competition in May. The song was in Italian, and she scored ninety-five out of one hundred which translated to a score of an "A". Level six was much more difficult, as the song choices were limited and most were in Italian. Megan works so hard at her craft, and she continues to improve and make wonderful progress.

Summer came around again, and although we wanted to go to Washington, DC, or back to Knoebels, we decided to stay closer to home and go on some day trips as a family. We went into New York City and saw some sights. We went to Adventureland Amusement Park, rode the rides, and had many laughs. We went out in my parents' boat and spent the day at the beach. And we went out to a really nice local restaurant for a wonderful meal. We had a really good time together and would like to do something like that again next year.

In November 2013, I made another big decision. Since things were again calming down in my life and I didn't already have enough to do (ha ha), I decided that I was finally going to start selling my homemade holiday cookies. I've been baking them for years to give as gifts and bringing them to work for all to enjoy. Every year, people tell me that I should open a bakery or sell the cookies somehow. When I did my baking the year before, in 2012, I took pictures of my different cookies and did some ground-work so that if I decided to sell them at some point, I would have something to show people.

I broke my recipes down by ingredients and estimated how many cookies each batch made. I then combined all of the ingredients that I would need, to determine how much of each item I was going to need to buy in total. For example, I figured out how many cups of sugar were in a five-pound bag or how many teaspoons of vanilla were in a one-ounce bottle, and so forth.

I put together a catalog, took orders, and baked my butt off. In the end, I had a great time and everyone loved my cookies. I think I cleared a couple hundred dollars. It wasn't much of a profit for all of that work, but I hope that what I did in 2013 will enable this side business to grow over time and become something that I can really concentrate on once my girls are out of high school.

Megan has been making great progress with her cerebral palsy. At one of my dad's appointments with his chiropractor, they started talking about Megan. The doctor suggested we make an appointment for Megan to see him, so I scheduled one for the end of November. He told us that her legs were different lengths because her right hip (her bad leg) was not sitting correctly. He worked on her and actually made both of her legs the same length. Her gait and smoothness when she walks have improved, and she feels great. She is now seeing the chiropractor and a massage therapist on a regular basis, and they are working on loosening all of the muscles in her right leg and ankle. Our next challenge coming up very soon is determining whether Megan will be able to drive a car without any special accommodations.

Megan's singing is progressing as well. At the time of this writing, she's working on another level six piece (also in Italian) to perform at the 2014 NYSSMA solo competition. She has also been dabbling in mixing and recording music this year at school, and she really likes it. Her teacher says that she's very good at it. If you don't see Megan performing on stage in the future, she might be one of the masterminds on the soundboards.

Emma has joined the junior archery league again this year. She's shooting at fifteen yards with a goal to move to twenty yards. Her first night, she shot a 119. By the end of the nine week league she was shooting a 204. Not only did her team come in first place, but she also got a trophy for most improved girl in the fifteen yard league. She's gotten so much better. Who knows, maybe one day you'll see her competing in the Olympic Games!

Happy New Year—2013 is over! Nearly ten years have gone by since I was first diagnosed! Lookout, 2014, here I come!

2014

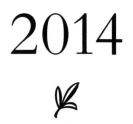

Chapter 72

Retrospective

In retrospect, what I went through in 2004 definitely changed my life. While "IT" impacted and changed the way I did things, I did not let "IT" define me. "IT" has actually made me a stronger person and made me realize how important my family is to me. I want my girls to see how my strength, my perseverance, and my love for them gave me the ability to make it through the toughest time in my life. I want Megan and Emma to be proud of me, and I want them to know how proud I am of them!

There are many different coping mechanisms and stress relievers that work differently for different people. One of my coping mechanisms was to feel like I had some control over part of my circumstances, so that I could come to terms with the things that I was unable to control. I also kept working, which was a very important mental aid to me. I rested when I felt tired or weak, which I hadn't really done prior to this experience. I started to realize what was important and what was not. I also decided that I wanted to put all of my extra energy into making my daughters' lives and experiences the best that they can possibly be.

As I sit here and finish writing this, I cannot believe that it has been ten years now since the beginning of the year that I would love to forget about. I know that no matter what, 2004 will always be a part of me. There will always be follow-up appointments to ensure that I continue to stay healthy. There will forever be new lumps and bumps that need to be looked at more closely. There will continue to be times when I start to overdo it and stretch myself too thin. I will have to rein myself back in and remember that I need to slow down, reduce my stress, and take some time for myself. Above all, I have learned that I have the right to be happy.

I sincerely hope that the information I've shared with you about my journey helps you in some way. Always stay positive, my friends!

Appendix A: My Quilt

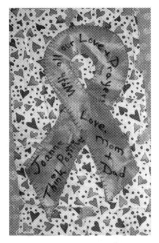

Mom and Dad

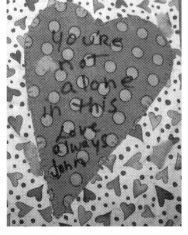

John

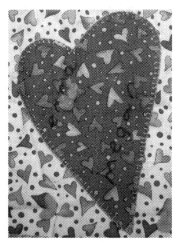

Megan and Emma

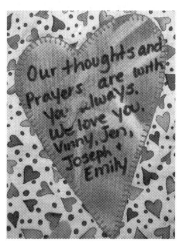

**Vinny, Jen, Joseph,
and Emily**

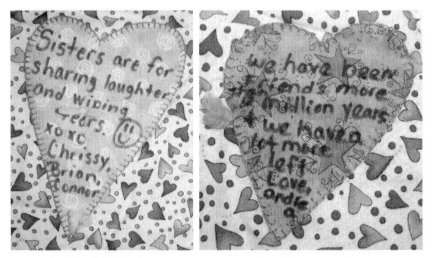

Chrissy, Brian, and Connor

Andrea

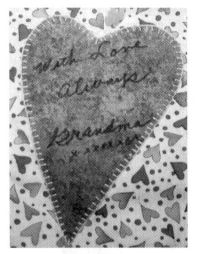

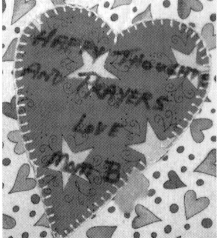

Grandma

Mom B

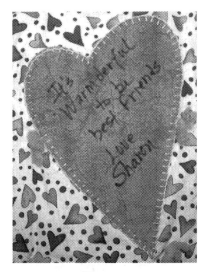

Sharon

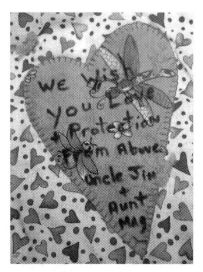

Aunt Maggie and Uncle Jim

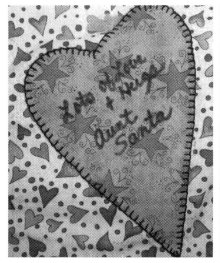

Aunt Santa

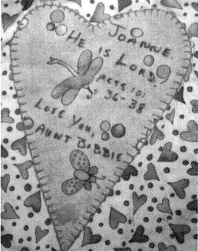

Aunt Barbara

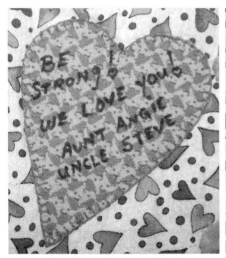

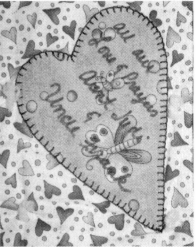

Aunt Angie and Uncle Steve   **Aunt Judy and Uncle Frank**

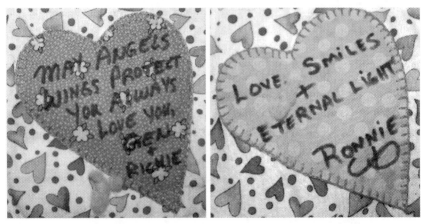

Gen and Richie   **Uncle Ronnie**

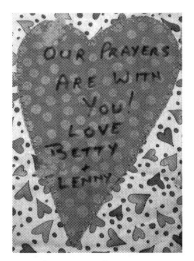

Betty and Lenny

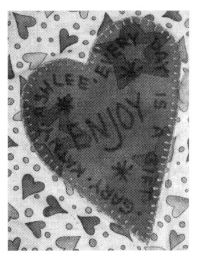

Kathy, Gary, and Ashlee

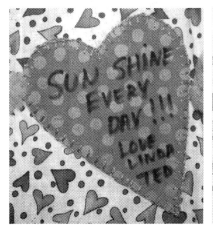

Linda and Ted

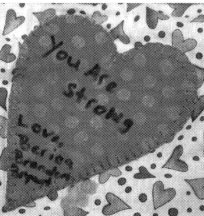

Berica, Brandon, and Bryant